Bearing of Basic Research on Clinical Otolaryngology

Advances in Oto-Rhino-Laryngology

Vol. 46

Series Editor
C.R. Pfaltz, Basel

KARGER

Basel · München · Paris · London · New York · New Delhi · Bangkok · Singapore · Tokyo · Sydney

Meeting of the Collegium Oto-Rhino-Laryngologicum Amicitiae Sacrum,
Basel, August 19–22, 1990

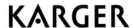
Bearing of Basic Research on Clinical Otolaryngology

Volume Editors
C.R. Pfaltz, Basel
W. Arnold, Luzern
O. Kleinsasser, Marburg

63 figures and 32 tables, 1991

KARGER

Basel · München · Paris · London · NewYork · New Delhi · Bangkok · Singapore · Tokyo · Sydney

Advances in Oto-Rhino-Laryngology

Library of Congress Cataloging-in-Publication Data
Collegium Oto-Rhino-Laryngologicum Amicitiae Sacrum. Meeting (1990: Basel, Switzerland)
Bearing of basic research on clinical otolaryngology / Meeting of the Collegium Oto-Rhino-Laryngologicum Amicitiae Sacrum, Basel, August 19–22, 1990;
volume editors, C.R. Pfaltz, W. Arnold, O. Kleinsasser.
(Advances in oto-rhino-laryngology; vol. 46)
Includes bibliographical references and index.
1. Labyrinth (Ear) – Diseases – Immunological aspects – Congresses.
2. Head – Tumors – Congresses.   3. Neck – Tumors – Congresses.
I. Pfaltz, C.R. (Carl Rudolf).   II. Arnold, W. (Wolfgang), 1941–.
III. Kleinsasser, O. (Oskar).   IV. Title.   V. Series.
[DNLM: 1. Head and Neck Neoplasms – congresses.
2. Labyrinth Diseases – immunology – congresses.
W1 AD701 v. 46 / WV 250 C697b 1991]
RF16.A38   vol. 46   [RF260]   617.5′1 s – dc20   [617.8′82]
ISBN 3–8055–5338–2

Bibliographic Indices
This publication is listed in bibliographic services, including Current Contents® and Index Medicus.

Contents

Preface

In the field of medical research a fundamental distinction should be recognized between medical research in which the aim is essentially diagnostic or therapeutic for the patient, and medical research the object of which is entirely scientific and primarily without any implication of diagnostic or therapeutic value to the person subjected to the research project. But in medicine both *basic* and *applied research* are linked together very closely and a major problem arises: the gap between *basic biomedical research* on the one side and the *application of its results* to human disease on the other. Unless this gap is bridged no further progress in medical diagnostics and therapeutics is feasible and for those reasons *clinical research* has to be promoted and developed. The point of departure and the goal of any *clinical research* is the human being, the patient.

In the office, at the hospital ward and in the operating theatre the scientifically minded physician is continuously confronted with problems exceeding the limits of a merely practically oriented medicine both diagnostically and therapeutically. These problems concern the cause, i.e. *etiology* and *pathogenesis*, of a *disease*, the *efficacy* of a medical or surgical *treatment*, the *causal factors* of *success* or *failure in therapy*. Clinical research is a continuing process integrated in the professional i.e. clinical activity of a physician or surgeon.

Prerequisites are an analytic mind, a scientific approach to methodology and above all a very high ethical standard as well as a strong sense of responsibility. We have to keep in mind that the scientist who is involved in clinical research may be daily confronted with the decision to transfer the knowledge gained experimentally in the laboratory to the human species. This transfer is part of an applied research methodology. This task demands a high scientific standard of the physician involved in clinical research and because of the great conceptional and technical advances in biomedical science a continuing education. There is every indication that such advances will continue to develop at an increasing rate. However, as science becomes more complicated, clinical scientists have greater difficulty in applying these advances to disease and basic scientists are needed. The complexity of disease-related problems forms a spectrum. Some of them exceed the ability of the traditional clinician to deal with them; others are less complex but necessitate collaboration between clinician and basic scientist.

The meeting of the Collegium Oto-Rhino-Laryngologicum Amicitiae Sacrum in Basel was an opportunity to promote communication between scientists active in the field of fundamental biomedical research and clinicians integrated in interdisciplinary research projects related with oto-rhino-laryngology. Recent advances in our understanding of cellular immunology, molecular biology and genetics have considerably influenced our approach to answer the riddle of the origin of idiopathic progressive perceptive deafness and of head and neck cancer. It was obvious that two major subjects should be chosen for a scientific presentation and discussion of the pending problems by competent representatives of fundamental and clinical research: (1) Immunobiology of inner ear diseases, and (2) Epidemiology, etiology and pathogenesis of head and neck cancer.

As an introduction to the theme – *The bearing of basic research on the investigation of clinical problems in otolaryngology* – W. Arber in his lecture of honour gave a brilliant state-of-the-art review of the advances in and the interdependence of molecular biology, genetic information, gene structure and biological functions.

The first symposium dealt with the major problem of *immune-mediated diseases of the inner ear*. W. Arnold moderated a sometimes controversial but very elucidatory panel discussion on immunological mechanisms underlying inner ear lesions. Special attention was paid to the question whether there really exists an *autoimmune disease in the inner ear*. Finally, the reliability of the various laboratory tests as well as the adequate treatment of cochleo-vestibular disorders, attributed to immune-mediated pathological involvement of the inner ear, were discussed in detail by competent scientists and clinicians.

The topic of the second symposium was selected because effective *prevention of head and neck cancer* needs a solid scientific basis, particularly with respect to *the role of extrinsic carcinogenic factors* such as tobacco, air pollution and nitrosamines *in combination with viral infections.* O. Kleinsasser moderated a highly interesting panel discussion in which competent scientists from important European cancer research institutes and cancer hospitals participated.

In conclusion, we may confirm that the original goal at which the founders of the Collegium ORLAS had been aiming has been reached: to invite a number of colleagues who take an interest in research in order to discuss fundamental scientific problems which are clinically relevant.

On behalf of the Board of the Collegium ORLAS, I should like to thank the Government of the Canton Basel-Stadt for taking over the official patronage of this international scientific meeting at the University of Basel and above all for offering a very generous subsidy of this publication.

Special thanks go also to the management of Ciba-Geigy Ltd. Basel for providing major support for the congress organization and to Dr. Thomas Karger for his substantial assistance.

Basel, August 1990   *C.R. Pfaltz*

Lecture of Honour

Pfaltz CR, Arnold W, Kleinsasser O (eds): Bearing of Basic Research on Clinical Otolaryngology. Adv Otorhinolaryngol. Basel, Karger, 1991, vol 46, pp 1–7

Contemplations on Genes and Biological Functions

Werner Arber

Biozentrum, University of Basel, Switzerland

Since the demonstration by Avery, MacLeod and McCarty in 1945 that DNA is the carrier of genetic information and since the publication by Watson and Crick in 1953 of the double-helix model of DNA, one has observed a rapid progress in the knowledge on gene structure and functions.

As in our written language, genetic information represents a linear sequence of letters, called nucleotides, of which only four different ones are used. In the double-stranded form, in which the juxtaposed letters are complementary, it is the nucleotide pairs which are linearly arranged, but because of the complementarity, it suffices to know the sequence of nucleotides in the so-called information strand.

The very long filamentous DNA molecules are replicated semiconservatively, i.e. each parental strand serves as a master in the synthesis of a new strand, a process which insures a high degree of fidelity in the transmission of the genetic information to daughter cells.

The total genetic information of an organism forms its genome. The information content per genome is quite high. The genomes of bacteria are composed of about 4×10^6 nucleotide pairs, about as many as the letters forming the Bible. The diploid genome of a human being contains about 6×10^9 nucleotide pairs, which one can compare with a library of about 1,500 volumes. Individual genes, the functional units of the genetic information, vary in length roughly between 100 and a few thousand letters. This corresponds to a few lines and one page of the library, respectively.

Note that a DNA molecule in isolation, outside of a living cell, is like a closed book, and an isolated genome can be compared to a locked library: nothing happens. It is only in a living cell that genes, by their carefully controlled expression, serve as the promoters of life activities. One can thereby distinguish between reading frames and control sequences. It is the latter's role to control when, where and with what intensity any particular biological function shall be turned on. Such functions usually are the consequence of the synthesis of one or a few gene products, mostly proteins. It is the reading frames, specific nucleotide sequences on the DNA, which serve as information transmitters in the synthesis of proteins. Since some proteins specifically interact with control sequences of the DNA and thus regulate the expression of other genes, the regulation of gene expression in a cell appears as a complex process with many interdependences of each particular gene from others.

Although genetic information is quite stable, mutations do occur spontaneously. These are alterations in the sequences of nucleotides. Mutations should not be considered as mistakes, rather they play a key role in the biological evolution. Many different mechanisms are known to contribute to spontaneous mutagenesis. Their action ranges from the simple substitution of one nucleotide by another to major rearrangements of the nucleotide sequences in the genome.

Classical genetic investigations always start with the isolation of mutants. Their altered phenotypic manifestation sometimes can already reveal the function of the affected gene. This strategy also has its importance in recent molecular genetic investigations, in which a gene of unknown function is often submitted to site-directed mutagenesis, a more straightforward approach than the classical random mutagenesis. However, site-directed mutagenesis relies on the knowledge of the nucleotide sequence of a gene.

Molecular genetics has its origins in microbial genetics developed in the last 50 years, particularly in the genetics of bacteria and their viruses and plasmids.

One interesting result of microbial genetics is the discovery of restriction enzymes. Such enzymes are produced by most bacterial strains. Their role is in the defence against foreign DNA invading a bacterium. Such invasion can be brought about by a number of different natural mechanisms. In transformation, free DNA molecules penetrate into a bacterial cell. In conjugation a plasmid, i.e. a short, independently propagated DNA molecule, serves as mediator and gene vector in the transmission of genetic information from one strain of bacteria to another. In transduction, it is a viral particle which serves as a vector for the transfer of cellular DNA to a new host cell of the virus. In any of these processes restriction enzymes not only recognize the invading DNA molecules as foreign, they also cut these DNA molecules in fragments, which represents an efficient step in their inactivation. Some restriction enzymes cut the DNA reproducibly within specific nucleotide sequences. These enzymes now serve as tools in research in that they cut the very long filaments of DNA into short specific fragments, thus making them accessible to molecular analysis, in particular sequence analysis and, as already mentioned, site-directed mutagenesis, an important approach in functional analysis.

While restriction fragments obtained from viral DNA can readily be purified, for example by gel electrophoresis, a high degree of purification is more difficult to reach with fragments of cellular genomes, because of a large number of different DNA fragments of often similar size. In vitro recombination helps to overcome this problem. In this technique, one DNA fragment is sorted out of a large population, then recombined with a vector DNA molecule, which can be the genome of a virus or a plasmid. This allows one to multiply the considered DNA segment as part of an autonomously replicating DNA molecule in appropriately chosen host cells. After reisolation of the multiplied DNA molecule the inserted DNA segment can be recovered and further analyzed. In this way molecular genetic techniques can be applied to any chosen cellular genetic information; hence structure and eventually also functions of any gene can be explored.

It is good to keep in mind that in vitro recombination usually implies the transfer of roughly one page out of the library of the genome of an organism into the genome library of another organism. Depending on the genetic content of the transferred DNA, the acquisition is or is not tolerated. The latter is the case if the functional harmony in the recipient cell becomes disturbed by the acquisition made.

However, the acquisition of small DNA segments is usually tolerated. This is in direct analogy with the already mentioned natural gene acquisition upon transformation, conjugation or virus-mediated transduction, in which restriction barriers cut the invading DNA into short segments, the occasional integration of which into the genome of a recipient cell is not only easily tolerated, but can also represent an important natural step in the biological evolution of the concerned microorganism. Similarly, in vitro recombination also represents a step in biological evolution – in this case of course under direct human influence. Risk assessment of recombinant DNA strategies will thus among others have to rely on our knowledge on the mechanisms of biological evolution.

The methodology of molcular genetics has already revealed many interesting aspects in the functioning of genes and their expression. Often, genes responsible for products involved in a particular biological pathway are coordinately expressed. This can be brought about by the juxtaposition of the concerned reading frames, so that the expression of the involved genes is controlled by the same control sequences, as it is best known for prokaryotic operons. Alternatively, the same regulatory protein(s) can control the expression of several genes located in various regions of the genome, if these genes are provided with the appropriate specific regulatory signals able to interact with the proteins in question.

It has become more and more evident that each control element has its characteristic efficiency and that control is not an all-or-none phenomenon. Rather, one often sees alternative expression to occur, which leads to the coordinate expression of from case to case more or less extended DNA sequences. This situation gives to the operon concept a qualitative rather than a quantitative nature. Alternative splicing of mRNA molecules (the intermediates between DNA and proteins in gene expression) is a similar process relying on probabilities rather than on strictly controlled mechanisms, by which segments of genetic information of a gene are brought together, while the gene as carried on the DNA represents a kind of mosaic structure containing irrelevant nucleotide sequences interspersed between functionally relevant sequences. In other systems, such as the immune systems of vertebrates, it is the gene segments on the DNA level that undergo rearrangements in the process of differentiation, hence functionality is here only assured in the differentiated lymphocytes. This process is also to some degree aleatoric and by far not all recombinations result in functional sequences. Interestingly, this process has much in common with evolutionarily relevant DNA rearrangements, which, as we have already seen, contribute to spontaneous mutagenesis.

These considerations obviously indicate that processes in the living world are often far from being perfect, as judged from the point of view of the investigator. Fidelity is quite high, as already said, in the replication of DNA. It is far less good in the production of RNA and it is relatively poor in the production of proteins. All of this can make sense. Indeed it mostly does not matter if a polypeptide does not take on a functional form, as long as there are other molecular products of the same gene which become functional. Usually nonfunctional products do not cause great harm and can thus be tolerated.

Despite of all the advances in molecular biology, it remains difficult to give a general definition of a biological function. To illustrate this point, one can ask if it is possible to construct a novel biological function in the laboratory. For the time being, this is not possible. There exists no biological theory allowing one to predict if a particular sequence of nucleotides determines a specific biological function. The question raised would have to be answered experimentally. Technically a nucleotoide sequence of the length of 1,000 nucleotides can be synthesized either according to a specific plan or at random. To study its functional potential, the synthetic DNA could be inserted into a genome and the recipient cell could be screened for an altered phenotype, which would indicate the functional relevance of the novel sequence. However, if such a test in for example *Escherichia coli* bacteria would be negative, it could still be possible that a function might be exerted in another organism, perhaps in spinach or in a cat. It will be very difficult to test all of the wide variety of potential host organisms. Another difficulty resides in the very great number of 10^{602} of possible different sequences to construct with 1,000 nucleotides. One can calculate that nature including all organisms that have lived up to today could at the very most have tested up to now 10^{50} different such sequences for their function. An experimental random approach to look for a novel biological function may appear hopeless in this situation.

We thus conclude that many imaginable applications of gene technology belong to science fiction and encounter serious natural limitations. Let us illustrate this with the following hypothetical example: In view of some of our sensory organs, such as the ear, which receives and converts sound waves into perception, and the eye, which receives electromagnetic waves of a certain wave-length and also converts them into perception – in both cases of course together with the brain – one could be tempted to construct the genes for an inbuilt receptor for radiowaves. Such a novel organ could act as a biological radio. Possibly several dozens or several hundreds of genes would be needed. But there is not the slightest indication available on how such gene sequences should look like. As we have already discussed, a random approach is most unlikely to be successful. Hence it is as unlikely that the genetic engineer could construct a completely novel living being. All he can do is to start with available genetic information on known biological functions and to attempt to produce alterations such as to improve or to delete a particular function. One also may try to transfer a particular function to other organisms. These strategies precisely correspond to what nature does all the time and what represents a motor of biological evolution. There is one difference however, processes of natural evolution are not directed towards a particular goal, while the genetic engineer may do so at least to some degree.

Let us direct our attention again to the natural strategies of biological evolution. By a steady development of the genetic information in a genome the population of the concerned organisms may slowly improve the genetic potential under the action of positive selection. This occurs mainly by alteration of existing functions, but to some degree also by the occasional appearance of a new function. All living species are submitted to this kind of genetic plasticity. Hence it clearly represents to living organisms an interesting alternative way to come to a new biological function, if occasionally developed novel functions can become transferred to other species. This is precisely what happens in natural gene acquisition, as it has already been discussed. Hence the randomly occurring acquisition is an efficient way to enrich a genome with a new functional potential in a single step. Because of the effects of reproductive isolation and of restriction systems, acquisition is tolerated to occur only rarely and in addition only in small steps. Only one or a few genes are usually acquired at once. This strategy ensures that by acquisition the functional harmony of the recipient cell has only a low probability to get disturbed. Needless to state that the success of acquisition benefits from the universality of the genetic code.

In view of the importance attributed to gene acquisition we draw the evolutionary tree as a network. In addition to the classical branching in this tree, horizontal shunts between the branches represent the possibilities of gene acquisition. Although acquisition occurs relatively rarely and in small steps its efficiency is high, much higher than that of the internal development of a new biological function in the vertical flux of a genome from generation to generation.

Some biologists consider biological evolution to be the result of accumulated errors. In this model spontaneous mutations are largely attributed to mistakes. Other biologists rather postulate that particular biological functions promote spontaneous alterations in the genetic message. In the latter in my opinion more correct model, biological evolution largely depends on enzyme activities, which act as variety generators. A number of different enzymes have been shown to exert such activities upon interaction with the DNA. In addition, natural gene vectors also may represent organelles with functions primarily serving the needs of biological evolution in that they promote gene acquisition.

Hence one can broadly classify biological functions into two groups. Biological functions of the first group meet the needs of individual lives. These genes are expressed at an appropriate level in each organism at the right time and at the right location. These are the gene products usually studied by biochemists and which catalyze largely reproducible reactions. Members of the second group of biological functions rather serve evolutionary needs. These functions are relatively rarely expressed. Although the genes coding for these functions are part of the genomes, their products are not relevant for each individual living organism. Rather, these biological functions are relevant at the population level, in that they contribute to increase genetic variety, which, on the other hand, is steadily reduced by the effect of natural selection. Without a constant, aleatoric replenishment of genetic variation, biological evolution could hardly be imagined to function properly. The broad classification given here for biological functions may appear to be too strict. Some biological functions may indeed serve both purposes, one to fill the needs of individual lives and the other to promote biological evolution. But some particular biological functions are likely to have been selected for in the course of time by their contributions made to biological evolution, rather than by having given immediate advantage to individual members of populations.

The opinion formulated here has its philosophical aspects and it may be of relevance with regard to our attitude towards life. It is somewhat unexpected that some of our genes may not function for a purpose of our own individual lives, but would exert their functions at the level of large populations. If such functions follow the strategy to generate genetic varieties and this not in a way directed to a particular goal, we will have to accept that a majority of the rare individuals experiencing the activity of such a biological function may as a matter of fact suffer from the consequences, since many spontaneous mutations are either lethal or of disadvantage. Rather rarely, mutations provide a selective advantage, and it is this latter category which provides evolutionary progress. In this view, genetic defects are not seen as errors, but rather as unavoidable products of the natural struggle to preserve and perpetuate life on the planet under steadily changing living conditions.

Werner Arber, MD, Professor of Microbiology, Biozentrum, University of Basel, Klingelbergstrasse 70, CH–4056 Basel (Switzerland)

Immunobiology of Inner Ear Diseases

Introduction

As early as 1958, Lehnhardt speculated that cases of progressive or fluctuating sensorineural hearing loss were due to 'allergic' mechanisms. Attempts at creating animal models of an immune mediated labyrinthitis were first performed by Beickert (1961), Terayama and Sasaki (1963), nearby in Freiburg. In 1974, Quick and Duvall as well as Arnold, Weidauer and Seelig (1975) demonstrated that an experimentally induced antibasement membrane glomerulonephritis – called Masugi nephritis – causes identic changes of the basement membranes of the stria vascularis, a possible model for Alport's syndrome.

McDonald and co-workers in 1978 reported cases of Alport's syndrome where the severe hearing loss improved dramatically after successful kidney transplantation. This might be caused either by the restored renal function or by the simultaneous immunosuppressive therapy. Improvement of hearing in Alport's syndrome means that there is no definitely fixed inner ear damage and that the state of cochlear function must be either directly related to the specific disease of the kidney or it is mediated by immunological factors.

With the clinical report of McCabe in 1979, further attention was focused on the possibility that certain forms of 'idiopathic' or 'cryptogenetic' sensorineural hearing loss are subject to an autoimmune pathomechanism. McCabe introduced the term 'autoimmune inner ear disease' although no conclusive proof was offered at that time. But it is due to McCabe, who stimulated researchers from all over the world to work experimentally and clinically in this field, that such fascinating data are available today. One most important result for example is the evidence of certain immunologic properties of the endolymphatic sac and its influence on the inner ear.

This symposium is devoted to a clarification of the state of the art and establishing perhaps a line along which future work can safely proceed.

W. Arnold

Pfaltz CR, Arnold W, Kleinsasser O (eds): Bearing of Basic Research on Clinical
Otolaryngology. Adv Otorhinolaryngol. Basel, Karger, 1991, vol 46, pp 9–16

Immunopathology and Autoimmunity:
The View of an Immunopathologist

F. Gudat

Institute of Pathology, University of Basel, Switzerland

This paper will focus on the basic immunopathological effector mechanisms in autoimmunity with special reference to possible manifestations
in the inner ear. Several criteria may be postulated to classify a disease as
autoimmune (table 1).

The *identification of the incriminated autoantigen* includes extraction
from normal tissue and characterization by immunochemical methods
such as Western blot or other appropriate tests as well as the demonstration of the autoantigen in situ by immunohistochemical methods in normal and diseased states.

The *demonstration of the specific immune mediators at the site of the
lesion,* i.e. immunoglobulin and complement components, is compelling
evidence. However, there are several drawbacks with current immunohistochemical techniques, particularly when working with the inner ear
embedded in bone tissue. The ideal processing of the tissue would require
shock-freezing in the native state and working on frozen sections. Even
then, the demonstration of immunoglobulins does not prove that they are
directed against the incriminated autoantigen. This could be shown only
with anti-idiotype antibodies tailored for the specific antigen-binding site
of the autoantibody. This and the need for fixation followed by decalcification makes this approach almost impossible at the present time. The
usual fixation with formalin and similar fixatives may cause reduction of
antigenicity, increased background staining and, most importantly, non-
immunologic fixation of free immunoglobulins to tissue components.
Often rather drastic enzymatic treatment of the sections has to be employed to unmask the antigenic site and to reduce background staining.
The simultaneous demonstration of individual complement components

Table 1. Definition of autoimmune disease

Essential criteria	Inconclusive criteria
Identification of the autoantigen	Demonstration of autoreactive lymphocytes and/or autoantibodies
Demonstration of (specific) immune mediators at the site of the lesion	Favorable response to immunosuppression
Proof of the primary pathogenicity	

such as C2, C4, C3 or the terminal membrane attack complex C5-9 would corroborate the interpretation of an immunologically relevant antigen-antibody interaction. It has to be borne in mind, however, that one frequently finds depots of immunoglobulins with or without complement within basement membranes and the interstitial tissue not associated with histopathologic or clinical signs of disease. As an example Alport's syndrome (hereditary nephritis) may be cited, an inherited progressive renal disease usually associated with nerve deafness. The glomerular lesion is due to the formation of an abnormal basement membrane. As disease progresses a secondary trapping of Ig/complement can be observed. Particularly mesangial accumulations of granular material without inflammation is seen also in many other degenerative states of the glomerular filter. Unfortunately, we have no reliable immunohistochemical markers at hand to identify biologically active immune complexes. On the other hand, deposition of otherwise inactive complexes into the basement membrane may cause functional holes without inflammatory reactions as evidenced by ongoing proteinuria.

The *demonstration of specific autoreactive T and/or B lymphocytes* would prove immunization against self – provided the autoantigen preparation used for in vitro stimulation is free of polyclonal stimulators. The same holds true for autoantibody determination – provided the test substrate, usually sections of the inner ear, is free of nonspecific binding which is likely to occur on fixed, decalcified sections. Even then, a positive autoimmunization does not necessarily prove a pathogenic involvement in the actual tissue damage. Many antitissue antibodies, particularly those against intracellular antigens, are not tissue-toxic and the sequel rather than the cause of a tissue lesion.

A *favorable response to immunosuppression* is in favor of an immunologically mediated disease but not proof of autoimmunity per se. To estab-
lish *primary autoimmune pathogenicity,* an exogenous tissue damage has
to be excluded and as many criteria in favor of autoimmunity as possible
have to be brought together. Other auxiliary criteria are association with
certain HLA-DR types, familial atopy, IgA immunodeficiency, complement deficiencies, age and sex [for review, see 1].

Once autoimmunity is established, as outlined by Melchers in this
volume, the immunologically mediated tissue damage can be assigned to
one or more of the classical hyperergic-allergic reaction types I–IV as
defined by Coombs and Gell [2].

Almost any organ may be involved as part of a multiorgan involvement (the inner ear, for instance, in polyarteritis nodosa) or it may be
affected in a organ-specific manner. In the latter case autoantigens of the
affected organ are both cause and target of the autoimmune response. Different forms of immune reaction may be anticipated depending on
whether the antigen is fixed on cells or tissue components or freely soluble
within the extracellular space or in fluids. With the most probable exception of allergic encephalitis and related multiple sclerosis, autoimmune
reactions are mediated by antibody and *not* by effector T cells. Therefore,
we shall concentrate on hyperergic-allergic types which are elicited by the
interaction of antibody with its target antigen.

Type I Reactions

As shown in table 2, type I reaction is specifically mediated by IgE in
concert with mast cells and their mediators in patients sensitized against
exogenous allergens such as pollen, house dust, etc. Since the inner ear is
not accessible for exogenous allergens and since, so far, there is no known
type I allergy against autoantigens, this type can be omitted from the
present discussion.

Type II Reactions

Type II reactions, i.e. interaction of autoantibody with tissue-bound
antigens (table 3), are predestined for organ-specific autoimmunity. Multiorgan involvement, however, is possible on the basis of shared cross-

reactivity. It is important to realize that it matters whether living cells or insoluble intercellular components such as basement membranes are involved and whether the autoantibody is capable to activate complement.

If surface antigens of living cells are the target, cell death, functional stimulation or blockade may ensue.

Two different cytotoxic reactions have been recognized. Activation of the complement cascade up to the formation of the terminal membrane attack complex formed by fragments of C5-9 may lead to *complement-mediated cell lysis*. The classical example for this is antibody-mediated hemolysis or lysis of other blood cells. As the term 'one-hit' theory indicates, this is a highly effective cytotoxic mechanism. However, nucleated cells may be resistant to this type of lysis and other mechanism may take

Table 2. The hyperergic-allergic reaction types of Coombs

	Antigenic properties	Specific mediators	Nonspecific mediators	Onset of reaction	Autoimmune disease
Type I	notself 'allergens'	IgE	mast cell eosinophil		unknown
Type II	notself e.g. viral	IgM IgG			immune hematology
	self cell surfaces basement membrane		complement macrophage mast cell	immediate	Goodpasture syndrome
Type III	notself e.g. viral self soluble self-components	IgM IgG IgA	(properdin)		immune complex diseases, e.g. lupus nephritis
Type IV	notself cell membrane-associated antigens self?	T lymphocytes	macrophage (epithelioid) NK cell	delayed	multiple sclerosis?

over. Opsonization of cells with IgG may lead to binding of Fc-receptor bearing macrophages and/or of natural killer cells which then are triggered to *antibody-derived cellular cytotoxicity* without the need of complement activation. Once necrosis is achieved, nonspecific inflammatory mechanism can then be recruited to remove damaged cells. An alternate consequence of antibody binding to cells has been detected in autoimmune endocrine diseases. Interaction with receptors on the cell surface may *block* the physiological role of the receptor as seen in myasthenia gravis or may *stimulate* the cell in place of the physiological ligand as found in immune thyrotoxicosis.

In the case of autoantibody fixation to basement membranes or other acellular tissue structures, necrosis is obviously not the primary damage. This is brought about, however, by activation of the complement cascade which generates secondary inflammatory mediators at each step leading to hyperemia, degranulation of mast cells and chemotaxis for granulocytes and macrophages. The classical experimental and naturally occurring example for this is antibasement membrane glomerulonephritis (Masugi nephritis and Goodpasture syndrome, respectively). In this condition, a linear deposition of IgG and complement components can be demon-

Table 3. Type II reactions ('cytotoxic type')

Subtype	Helper system	Pathogenesis	Possible target in inner ear	Autoimmune analogue
Cytotoxic			basement membrane collagens	autoimmune hemolytic anemia
(a) AB + complement mediated	complement	activation of complement	hair cells epithelial and mesothelial cells	
(b) AB mediated cellular cytotoxicity	Fc-bearing NK cells and macrophages	killing via cell-to-cell contact		?
Blocking	none	steric blockade of receptor	hair cells nerve cells	myasthenia gravis
Stimulating	none	stimulation of receptor	?	autoimmune hyperthyroidism

strated along the glomerular basement membrane. This is accompanied by infiltration with neutrophils and often also by activation of the coagulation system leading to crescent formation of Bowman's capsule with a high probability of obliteration of the glomerulus. Interestingly, a glomerular basement membrane antigen has been shown to cross-react with the stria vascularis in the guinea pig [3]. Even in the absence of severe inflammatory damage there might be a structural alteration of the basement membrane causing increased permeability which by itself may cause proteinuria and erythruria.

Type III Reactions

Complex formation between freely soluble antigen and autoantibody with or without activation of complement is very common in autoimmune disease. Obviously, this type is particularly prone to multiorgan involvement since immune complexes may circulate in the body and may be deposited in primarily unrelated organs. Basement membranes and filter organs are predilection sites. Once complexes are deposited, they may be modulated by apposition and/or dissolution depending mainly on the relative amount (antigen or antibody excess) and quality of the antibody

Table 4. Type III reactions ('immune-complex type')

Subtype	Helper system	Pathogenesis	Possible target in inner ear	Autoimmune analogue
IgM, IgG$_1$, IgG$_2$, IgG$_3$	clotting system	activation of complement ± clotting system	stria vascularis basement membranes	immune complex vasculitis immune complex nephritis
	macrophages leukocytes mast cells	mast cell degranulation		
IgA, IgG$_4$	properdin (alternate pathway)			

(antibody class, affinity, charge). Other factors are size and charge of the antigen and local microenvironment.

This complicated interplay is best illustrated by glomerulonephritis of the immune-complex type (table 4). Depending on the quality of the complexes one might find a deposition in subendothelial, intramembranous or epimembranous location. In addition, it is well known that the size of IgM or IgA complexes favors deposition in the subendothelial and mesangial space, along the natural pathway for clearance of macromolecules which are excluded by the basement membrane.

Type IV Reactions

Whereas the T lymphocyte plays a key role in the regulation of autotolerance and autoaggression, its role as an effector cell in autoimmunity is less apparent. However, multiple sclerosis as the best accepted model for T cell-mediated lysis of myelinated nerve cells should alert us that nerve cells of the inner ear might become a target for autoreactive T effector cells.

Inner Ear and Autoimmunity

Preconditions for an immunologically mediated reaction in the inner ear are well described. Within the region of the endolymphatic sac the cellular and humoral components (lymphocytes, plasma cells, mast cells and immunoglobulins, respectively) have been demonstrated, probably representing part of the mucosa-associated lymphoid tissue [4]. Experimentally, using inner ear tissue, autoimmunity could be produced [Harris, this volume].

Based on the outlined immunopathological reaction types one would expect cytotoxic type II reactions preferentially with hair cells, epithelial and mesothelial cells, whereas immune complex-mediated type III reactions are particularly likely to occur as part of a more generalized form in the stria vascularis and in basement membranes involved in filter function. The degree of inflammation and destruction is modulated by the recruitment of nonspecific cellular and humoral systems such as mast cells, macrophages, granulocytes as well as the complement and the clotting system. Immunohistochemistry could be very helpful to identify these specific and nonspecific components in autoimmunity.

References

1   Coombs RRA, Gell PGH: Classification of allergic reactions responsible for clinical hypersensitivity and disease; in Gell PGH, Coombs RRA, Lachmann PJ (eds): Clinical Aspects of Immunology, ed 3. Oxford, Blackwell Scientific, 1975, pp 761–781.

2   Shoenfeld Y, Isenberg DA: The mosaic of autoimmunity. Immunol Today 1989;10: 123–126.

3   Arnold W, Weidauer H, Seelig HP: Experimenteller Beweis einer gemeinsamen Antigenizität zwischen Innenohr und Niere. Arch Otorhinolaryngol 1976;212:99–117.

4   Arnold W, Altermatt HJ, Gebbers JO: Qualitativer Nachweis von Immunoglobulinen im menschlichen Saccus endolymphaticus. Laryng Rhinol Otol 1984;63:464–467.

Prof. Dr. F. Gudat, Institute for Pathology, University of Basel,
Schönbeinstrasse 40, CH–4003 Basel (Switzerland)

Pfaltz CR, Arnold W, Kleinsasser O (eds): Bearing of Basic Research on Clinical
Otorhinolaryngology. Adv Otorhinolaryngol. Basel, Karger, 1991, vol 46, pp 17–25

Immunity and Autoimmunity

With Special Reference to Inner Ear Diseases

Fritz Melchers

Basel Institute for Immunology, Basel, Switzerland

*The Diverse Repertoire of Antigen Recognizing Lymphocytes Has the
Potential to be Autoantigen-Reactive*

The antigen-recognizing repertoire of T cell receptors (TcR) on T lymphocytes and antibody (Ig) molecules on B lymphocytes is potentially
autoantigen-reactive. This must be so because TcR and Ig genes are generated during the development of lymphocytes from stem cells and progenitors by rearrangements of multiple V, D and J (TcR β and δ, Ig H chain
genes), respectively V and J segments (TcR α and γ, Ig L chain genes),
superimposed by additional variabilities of N-sequences generated in the
gene segment-joining processes at the junctions of V, D and J.

The diversity of variable (V) regions of TcR and Ig with the three
complementary-determining regions (CDR) making contact with an antigen is, therefore, expected to be so great that at least one of the 10^{12} lymphocytes in the immune system of man will be able to bind to a given
chemical structure – and that, therefore, *any* structure within or without
the system can be bound by one of these lymphocytes.

Since one lymphocyte expresses only one TcR or one Ig, i.e. generated
by *one* (of millions and millions) unique sets of rearrangements in TcR α
and β, or γ and δ genes, or in Ig H and L chain genes, some of the lymphocytes are expected to be autoreactive, others not. Furthermore, it appears
that selected sets of V_γ/V_δ combinations – and maybe even some V_α/V_β sets
– of TcR are autoantigen-binding not because of their accidental variabil-

ity generated by the joining process (and therefore expressed in the structure of the third CDR), but because the first and second CDRs of some V-segment gene sequences inherit self-recognition in the germ line. As one example, certain α/β TcR sets with very little or no N-region diversity appear to recognize transplantation (MHC) class I-related molecules. As another example, certain of α/β TcR combinations appear to be used by T cells which dominate T cell responses in autoimmune diseases such as rheumatoid arthritis or multiple sclerosis.

T Cell Tolerance

T cell progenitors entering the thymus are induced to rearrange their α, β, γ and δ TcR gene segments, and to express γ/δ or α/β TcR, each individual one on one T cell. This diverse repertoire is then subjected to positive and negative selection in the thymus. During *positive* selection, all T cells expressing a TcR capable of binding to MHC class I or II molecules (expressed on epithelial cells of the thymic stroma) are induced to survive, while all other T cells *not* fitting to these MHC molecules die. During *negative* selection, TcR-expressing T cells binding to MHC class I or II molecules on hematopoietic cells in the thymus (dendritic cells, macrophages) are induced to die. MHC class I and II molecules are expected to present processed autoantigens. Consequently, positive and negative selection includes all self antigens present in the thymus, whenever the processed peptides of those autoantigens fit into self MHC class I or II molecules. It is expected that the process of positive selection includes lower interactions of TcR with self MHC/auto peptides than the process of negative selection does, in order to allow T with less avid TcR to survive and enter the peripheral lymphoid compartment, where they appear 'MHC-restricted' in the recognition of *foreign* antigens. In summary, the thymus discards the useless, destroys the harmful and selects the (potentially) useful TcR repertoire of cytolytic and of helper T cells.

In the periphery, *foreign* antigens are processed and presented on self MHC molecules expressed on antigen-presenting dendritic cells, macrophages, B cells and possibly other MHC class I or II molecules. If the mature T cell repertoire contains a cell with a TcR fitting this combination of foreign peptide and self MHC better than self peptide with self MHC, this T cell is stimulated to a positive response of proliferation and maturation to effector functions. Recognition in the context of MHC class I leads to cytolytic T cells, in the context of MHC class II to helper T cells, which can either help B cells to proliferation and Ig secretion or induce inflammatory responses. T cells do not mutate their TcR genes in any way once they have left the thymus – and that safeguards them from possible changes of their antigen specificity toward autoreactions.

MHC Linkage of Diseases – Ig Genes

MHC class I and II genes are highly polymorphic. Different individuals express different MHC molecules, which have different capacities to bind given processed peptides of antigens. As a consequence, a given individual can be a high or a low responder to a given antigen, not because of a difference in the T cell repertoire but because of a difference in MHC molecules binding peptides. T cell responses to a given antigen are, therefore, genetically linked to a given MHC haplotype, probably because a disease-inducing or -propagating antigen (foreign or self) is either poorly or well bound to this given MHC molecule.

B Lymphocytes and Their Responses to Antigen

In contrast to T cells, B cells are not severely depleted of self-reactive cells, although their Ig-receptor repertoire appears to be potentially as diverse as that of T cells, with multiple V, D and J segments of the H chain gene locus and the multiple V and J segments of the L chain loci rearranging with N-region diversity to a very high number of different V_H/V_L combinations of Ig molecules. Although depletion, and also anergy, of autoreactive B cells have been observed during B cell generation from progenitor cells in fetal liver and bone marrow, it is easy to find autoantigen binding to Ig molecules produced, and upon stimulation, secreted by B cells. T cell-independent and polyclonal stimulations, however, do not lead to extensive somatic hypermutations of the Ig H and L chain genes, nor to extensive switching to other classes of Ig (IgG, IgA), and not to longer-lived B cells, and memory for the antigenic encounter. Many responders to foreign antigens are accompanied by the production of IgM-class (but not switched Ig classes) rheumatoid factors. Two types of autoantigens appear to be involved: DNA-protein complexes and Ig-Fc-receptors of antigen-specific antibodies (made in the response to foreign antigens). These rheu-matoid-IgM responses appear to be stimulated by repetitive determinants (of DNA, of Fc-receptors) cross-linking surface Ig or B cells specific for these autoantigens. This cross-linking may, in fact, *inhibit* the elicitation of T cell-dependent responses in such B cells, and thus, avoid the develop-ment of autoimmune diseases of rheumatoid types (see below). In order to induce memory, to induce hypermutation of the Ig genes, to induce class switching and to induce longer-lived B cells specific for the antigen, B cells have to be stimulated with the help of CD4-positive helper T cells. While T cell-independent antigens are thought to cross-link surface Ig as antigen-specific receptors and, thus, stimulate B cells regardless of their MHC haplotype, T cell-dependent antigens are often monovalent, are taken up by surface Ig of antigen-specific B cells and are then processed and pre-sented as peptides by MHC class II molecules on these B cells. This com-plex of processed antigen and self MHC class II molecules is then recog-nized by the TcR of helper T cells. T cell-dependent responses of B cells are, therefore, MHC-haplotype-restricted. As a consequence of this con-tact between TcR of T cells and MHC plus peptide on B cells, T cells produce cytokines which propagate the proliferation and maturation to Ig secretion, as well as class switching and hypermutation, of the activated B cells. Antigen then continues to select B cells with somatically mutated Ig receptors which have mutated to higher activity, i.e. bind the antigen bet-ter than before. In summary, selected, somatically mutated Ig specific for an antigen is taken as a hallmark of a helper T cell-dependent B cell response.

Such memory responses cannot develop to an autoantigen, *not* be-cause autoantigen-binding B cells do not exist to take up and present the antigen, but because the autoantigen-peptide/self MHC class II-specific helper T cells have been eliminated in the thymus.

Suppression

Suppression of immune responses are commonly observed in the immune system, and are thought to involve a variety of different mecha-nisms and cells. Autoantigen-specific suppression mediated by antigen-specific suppressor cells is, however, still a controversial area in immuno-logical research, primarily because clones of antigen-specific suppressor T cells are still not available for experimentation.

Breaking Tolerance

Our current understanding of the functioning of the immune system, its repertoires of antigen recognition, its regulation of the class of responses, and its distinction between autoantigens and foreign antigens ascribes the domineering role in the regulation to helper T cells, and the role in the distinction between 'self' and 'nonself' to helper T cells and cytolytic T cells. Therefore, in autoimmune diseases we search for abnormal interactions between helper T cells and antigen-presenting cells, guided by the interaction of TcR with antigenic peptides bound on MHC class II molecules, which lead to inflammatory responses and to autoantibody production of switched classes of Ig molecules. We search for abnormal cytolytic T cells interacting with their TcR, with antigenic peptides bound on the MHC class I molecules. The abnormal interactions are expected to lead to tissue destruction, wherever antibody (and antigen-antibody complexes) plus complement, or cytotoxic T cells against specific cells of the target tissue are involved.

Four major categories of 'abnormal' changes in T cell-antigen-presenting cell interactions, leading to autoimmune T cell activation, can be envisaged:

(1) Changes involving the uptake or synthesis, processing and presentation of antigen. Antigen may be hidden at immunologically nonaccessible sites (intracellular compartments, organs, such as brain with cellular barriers to blood), or might be encoded by genes which might become abnormally activated (abnormal expression of differentiation antigens, normally silent retroviral genes, stress proteins (heat shock), etc.). As long as these antigens were not presented to the thymus, it is likely that peripheral T cells exist which will be activated when these gene products appear.

The concentration of an autoantigen might be abnormally increased. The increase in concentration of processed autoantigen will allow binding to MHC with lower activity which, in turn, will activate hitherto resting T cells.

If a foreign antigen can form a covalently bound complex with an autoantigen (tanning reactions, drugs, other chemicals binding to epithelia etc.) monovalent binders uptake the processing of this complex by autantibody-producing B cells will allow their T cell-dependent activation, somatic hypermutation and class switching of their Ig genes by helper T cells recognizing the processed foreign antigen on MHC class II molecules of the B cells.

A foreign antigen can mimic an autoantigen in that both structures are bound by the same B cell. Processing and presentation by the foreign antigen, however, will generate a foreign peptide which is different from any peptide processed from the corresponding autoantigen. Therefore, T cells will exist in the mature repertoire which stimulate the B cell-producing Ig molecules with the capacity to recognize the foreign as well as the autoantigen. They then stimulate hypermutation and Ig class switching. If the somatic mutants selected by the foreign antigen bind also better to the autoantigen, mimicry is perfect – and autoimmune antibodies with higher avidities are selected by the foreign antigen. We know of several viral infections where such antigenic mimicry is suspected to be the cause for autoimmune disease.

(2) Changes in the expression of MHC antigens. MHC molecules on the surface of cells can change their level of expression. As one example, the expression of MHC class II molecules is up-regulated on antigen-presenting cells upon stimulating interaction with helper T cells. Cytokines such as IL-4 and γ-IFN produced by helper T cells are known to stimulate this up-regulation. A constitutive up-regulation of MHC molecules to higher than normal levels, and even in the absence of cytokine stimulation, is expected to lead to a positive response of hitherto resting cells with TcR of lower avidities to autoantigen peptides on MHC molecules.

MHC molecules (especially the less ubiquitously expressed class II molecules) might also become expressed by cells which normally do not do so. This may make these cells, and the sites of the body where they lodge, abnormally immunocompetent. Autoantigens confined to these sites might, therefore, become immunostimulatory.

(3) Changes in the expression of autoantigens and of MHC molecules in the thymus. If changes of autoantigen expression (especially to nonexpression) and MHC antigen (do different levels) occur in the thymus, or if the antigen-presenting functions during positive, and particularly negative selection, are deregulated at any other molecular or cellular level, a change in the T cell repertoire emerging in the periphery should result. This change might include the emergence of autoantigen-reactive T cells in the mature peripheral organs, which normally would have been deleted in the thymus.

(4) Transformation of T cells or antigen-presenting cells. The somatic mutation of genes involved in proliferation and/or effector functions of helper or cytolytic T cells leading to preneoplastic states of cellular performance, or similar changes in the compartment of antigen-presenting cells

are likely to have autoimmune disease-propagating effects, particularly if these changes occur in autoantigen-reactive T cells. Despite intensive investigations into the mechanism of T cell activation and T cell-antigen-presenting cell interactions, we have yet to define the proto-oncogenes which cause transformations to such preneoplastic states.

The deregulation of autoreactive γ/δ TcR-T cells, and of the elusive antigen-specific suppressor T cells, are other ways by which tolerance might be broken, but a reasonable discussion of these potential autoimmune attacks awaits a clarification of the nature and the normal functions of these cells.

In conclusion, it is easily conceivable that stepwise changes involving more than one of the ways by which tolerance can be broken could lead to an increase in the severity of autoimmune disease. In particular, combinations of abnormalities in the helper and in the cytolytic T cell compartments are likely to compound the autoimmune pathological effects of inflammation, antigen-antibody complexes plus complement, and T cell-mediated cytolysis. A continued analysis of the genetics of T cell responsiveness (HLA- and non-HLA- (minor antigens) linkage, etc.), and of general susceptibilities (proto-ontogenes, etc.), and of the epidemiology (infections, environmental influences (chemical drugs, etc.) begins to be able to uncover the lesions which lead to a given autoimmune disease, and to distinguish different ways by which one disease can develop. Ultimately, this should guide more differential treatment protocols of only apparently identical diseases.

Are Inner Ear Diseases Caused by Immune or Autoimmune Reactions?

A subgroup of sensorineural hearing losses (SNHL) is suspected to have immune, and maybe autoimmune, destruction of the inner ear as a cause. In particular, bilateral deafness with immune complex deposition on the epithelial cells of the endolymphatic sac of the inner ear, and a high frequency of cases of systemic lupus-like specificities of autoantibodies (ANA, smooth muscle, microsomes as antigens) in the endolymphatic fluid of the inner ear are such cases of SNHL. Although cortisone does not only effect lymphocyte growth and survival but has many other cellular targets, it is often used as an immunosuppressant and its effect to slow down and obliterate some cases of SNHL has been used as an argument for an immune or autoimmune cause of the disease.

A number of questions can be asked to evaluate the possible immuno-pathological origin of SNHL, and to find new ways for a differential immunosuppressive treatment of the disease.

(1) Is the inner ear capable of mounting normal, protective immune responses? Do parts of the inner ear have the characteristic structures (organization of tissue, cells, molecules) of a lymphoid organ? The inner ear is considered to be an extension of the central nervous system (CNS). Although CNS is shielded by the blood-brain barrier (as the inner ear is by the blood-labyrinthine barrier), and although Ig molecules and lymphocytes are found at one thousandth the concentration found in blood, these concentrations still appear to suffice for the elicitation of an immune response against unknown antigens in experimental allergic encephalomyelitis and in multiple sclerosis, which develop extensive immunopathological lesions in the brain. Lymphocytes and macrophages have been found in the endolymphatic sac and in the perisaccular tissue of experimentally nonstimulated tissue. Although a more thorough up-to-date analysis of the inner ear for the major players of an immune response (T cells, B cells, macrophages, dendritic cells, etc., with their characteristic markers and functions) is desirable, this current knowledge at least does not rule out that the endolymphatic sac is an organ capable of immune reactions.

Immune reactions in the inner ear have been experimentally elicited to foreign antigens by local administration. Local antibody production, distinct from CNS and blood, has been observed in primary and secondary responses, both by the production of antigen-specific 'switched' classes of Ig, as well as by the induction of inflammatory reactions in the scala tympani and within the perisaccular connective tissue and the endolymphatic sac. The obliteration of the endolymphatic sac before antigenic challenge leads to a marked reduction in the local specific antibody production. Protective immunity to *cytomegalovirus* has been observed in humans, but the primary route of infection is certainly not restricted to the inner ear, although the infection can lead to *labyrinthitis* and SNHL.

(2) What makes an immune response to the inner ear pathological? Primary, and particularly secondary, responses in animals against experimentally administered antigens can lead to SNHL. In SNHL of humans these questions then arise: (a) Is the response a defense against a foreign infectious agent on inner ear cells? (b) Is the response autoimmune, and directed against antigens of the inner ear? (c) Which are the antigens (autoantigens)? (d) Which cells in the inner ear are attacked? Are they

destroyed or incapacitated? (e) Is it a *local* response, or is it a 'bystander' response of a systemic response which passes the blood-labyrinthine barrier? (f) Are there several types of pathological immune responses, and can they be grouped into subtypes by genetics and epidemiology? Answers to these questions will hopefully guide better and more differentiated treatment protocols in a fight against at least some of the forms of inner ear destruction.

Prof. Fritz Melchers, PhD, Basel Institute of Immunology, PO Box,
CH–4005 Basel 5 (Switzerland)

Pfaltz CR, Arnold W, Kleinsasser O (eds): Bearing of Basic Research on Clinical
Otolaryngology. Adv Otorhinolaryngol. Basel, Karger, 1991, vol 46, pp 26–33

Experimental Immunology of the Inner Ear

Jeffrey P. Harris

Division of Otolaryngology, Department of Surgery, University of California,
San Diego Medical Center, and the Research Service,
Veterans Administration Medical Center, San Diego, Calif., USA

It has been slightly over 10 years since McCabe [1] first reported a treatable form of sensorineural hearing loss (SNHL) that appears to have an autoimmune basis. Since that time, studies have focused on the pathogenesis, diagnosis, and treatment of this disorder.

Evidence has since been accumulated which suggests that immune-mediated deafness is a distinct entity and that therapy with immunosuppressive agents is, in early cases, beneficial with regard to hearing. Unfortunately, no prospective controlled studies have been performed to date to investigate the optimal diagnostic criteria, nor the most efficacious form of treatment for this disease.

This paper will explore the histopathological and experimental data that currently exists to support immunological mechanisms responsible for SNHL.

Histopathology

There are limited examples of temporal bones from patients with immune-mediated deafness. In fact, no temporal bone findings from patients with the diagnosis of autoimmune SNHL have been reported to date. Rather, there have been sporadic reports of the temporal bone findings in patients with polyarteritis nodosa (PAN) and Cogan's syndrome. The histopathological features were reported by Gussen [2], who found arteritis in the internal auditory artery with widespread cochleovestibular ischemic changes, and osteoneogenesis and fibrotic tissue in the basilar turns. Jenkins et al. [3] reported similar pathologic findings, but these were restricted to the cochlea.

In a temporal bone study, Yanagita et al. [4] reported a case of bilateral deafness associated with nephritis and a B-cell lymphoma. In this patient, necrotizing vasculitis was seen in small- and medium-sized arteries throughout the body in association with PAN, and there was complete disappearance of the organ of Corti, atrophy or absence of the stria vascularis, collapse of Reissner's membrane, distortion of the tectorial membrane, as well as bone formation and fibrosis of the apical turn. Many of these findings have been experimentally produced by sudden interruption of cochlear blood flow [5, 6]. Thus, from the temporal bone findings, one can conclude that vasculitis is one clearly definable cause of profound hearing loss. In Cogan's syndrome, a condition of young adults characterized by nonsyphilitic interstitial keratitis and vestibuloauditory dysfunction [7–9], the temporal bone findings consist of endolymphatic hydrops, plasma cell and lymphocytic infiltration of the spiral ligament [10], saccular rupture, osteoneogenesis of the round window, spiral ganglion cell degeneration, and cystic degeneration of the stria vascularis [11]. In addition, Zechner [12] found degeneration of the organ of Corti, as well as fibrosis and osteoneogenesis within the perilymphatic space. In another temporal bone study, bilateral cochlear osteoneogenesis and ectopic bone tissue within the vestibule and semicircular canals were found in a patient with Cogan's syndrome [13].

At this symposium, Schuknecht [14] reports on the temporal bone findings of a patient with probable immune-mediated deafness and systemic eosinophilia. It seems clear, then, that inner ear immune processes result in histopathological changes that are characteristic and consistent with the observed alterations of inner ear function seen clinically. We still await, for comparison, the temporal bone findings from a patient with autoimmune SNHL, in whom there are no other systemic signs of autoimmunity.

Experimental Studies

Since the inner ear is inaccessible to study, much of what is known about immunity necessarily comes from animal models. These studies have attempted to elucidate whether the inner ear is a passive site, unable to participate in immune responses, or one which can mount immunological reactions that resemble those seen in other organs of the body, particularly the central nervous system (CNS), of which the inner ear is an extension. This is particularly germane since many of the degenerative or progressive diseases that affect the CNS are due in great part to the immune reactions occurring in those tissues [15]. In this regard, one must separate these responses into normal immunological responses as part of the host's normal defense mechanisms or autoimmune reactions in which the host's immune system is self-directed.

In both of these scenarios the organ involved, which in this instance is the inner ear, may become injured due to the deleterious effects of the inflammatory response. One occurs as a result of bystander injury while the other results from a specific immune response directed toward tissue components of the inner ear.

Early studies suggesting that the inner ear is not an immunoprivileged site come from the observation that immunoglobulin crosses the blood-labyrinthine barrier and is found in perilymph at a level of 1/1,000 of the concentration found in serum in a manner analogous to the blood-brain barrier [16, 17]. Increased concentrations of immunoglobulin are also seen within the perilymph relative to the cerebrospinal fluid (CSF) [16, 17]. It is unknown whether this is the result of the water-resorptive properties of the inner ear or a specific concentrative mechanism. The end result is an immunoglobulin-rich environment that must serve to protect the inner ear from pathogens. The immunoglobulin found in human and animal peri-lymph appear to be predominantly IgG, with lesser amounts of IgM and IgA identified [17, 18]. Arnold et al. [19] have demonstrated secretory component and IgA in the endolymphatic sac (ES) epithelial cells, suggest-ing that this site may be part of the mucosal immune system, an observa-tion which we have confirmed in our own laboratory [Takahashi and Har-ris, pers. observation].

The next step in assessing how such an immune system operates would be to stimulate the inner ear selectively with antigen. In a series of studies from our laboratory, we have challenged the perilymph of naive (primary response) and sensitized (secondary response) animals and observed the antibody levels developing in the perilymph over time. Results of these studies demonstrate that: (1) local production of antibody occurs in the inner ear; (2) secondary-response animals develop much higher antibody levels than primary response animals, and (3) these responses are indepen-dent of CSF or serum [20, 21].

The accumulation of inflammatory cells within the inner ear can be seen in response to many stimuli (infection, trauma, immunological reactions, or interruption of blood flow). This finding has been a regular observation in all of our studies to date, therefore, we questioned how these cells might enter the inner ear. By examining animals temporally, and as early as 6 h poststimulation, we began to see the accumulation of cells around and within the spiral modiolar vein, adjacent to the scalae tympani [21]. Furthermore, as these reactions developed, cells (PMNs, lymphocytes) began to stream into the scala tympani along the bony canaliculi containing the collecting venules. As time progressed, organization of these cells was often noted, resulting in fibrosis or osteoneogenesis. In the same study, we analyzed human temporal bones in which suppurative labyrinthitis was diagnosed and 15 ears showed the identical mechanism of cellular egress into the scala tympani via the spiral modiolar vein. These observations explain the propensity for fibrosis to develop preferentially within the scala tympani rather than the scala vestibuli, since the former is the venous side of the inner ear, and cells can only emigrate from systemic circulation via the venous system and not the arterial system.

The signal for such an event may be in a class of hormones known as interleukins (IL). These low molecular weight glycoproteins have multiple roles, including T and B cell activation and chemoattraction. We measured IL-2 in antigen-stimulated inner ears and found that the peak rise in perilymph IL-2 was at 18 h and declined over 5 days. This corresponds well with the accumulation of helper T cells and macrophages within the inner ear [22].

Since there must be resident cells within the inner ear that respond to antigen challenge, our next step was to examine sites where cells that can elaborate IL might be located. Because of the close interaction of lymphocytes and macrophages observed within the lumen, the ES has been suggested as the site of host defenses within the inner ear [23, 24]. Studies involving immunohistochemical analysis of the ES under normal and immunologically stimulated conditions have demonstrated that each of the cell populations required for immune processing exist in the normal sac and expand following stimulation [25, 26]. By 3 weeks, suppressor T cells which were absent in the unstimulated sac begin to appear, presumably to halt the inflammatory response. Further, to test the central role of the ES in these responses, experiments were performed in which the ES was surgically ablated prior to inner ear immune stimulation [27–29]. In these cases, there was a significant reduction of both antibody levels and inflammation in the sac-obliterated ears compared to the normal intact ear. This observation was confirmed independently by Morgenstern et al.

[30]. Subsequent studies blocking the endolymphatic duct and preserving the ES before antigen challenge of the scala tympani confirmed both the importance of the ES in the elaboration of the immune response and that this site represents the afferent limb for inner ear immunity [27, 28]. Thus, it seems that the ES provides an immunologic as well as water-resorptive role for the inner ear in a manner analogous to that of the gut, which is also known to serve both purposes.

The concept that the inner ear may also be the target of autoimmune conditions follows from extensive experimental studies conducted on other organ systems. Such animal models have been established for experimental allergic encephalomyelitis, allergic neuritis, myasthenia gravis, and allergic thyroiditis, to name a few. In 1961, Beickert [31] performed the first study to examine this possibility in relation to the inner ear. Using guinea pigs immunized to inner ear antigen, he was able to demonstrate lesions within the cochlea. In 1963, Terayama and Sasaki [32] immunized guinea pigs with isologous cochlear tissue in Freund's adjuvant and were also able to produce isolated lesions within the cochlea and alterations in Preyer's reflex. Neither study was able to document the development of anticochlear antibodies nor the presence of perivascular infiltrates. These observations were essentially ignored at that time.

Since then, Yoo et al. [33] have reported the development of an animal model with inner ear injury secondary to type II collagen autoimmunity. These animals demonstrated spiral ganglion cell degeneration, atrophy of the organ of Corti, arteritis of the cochlear nerve and stria vascularis, and endolymphatic hydrops with atrophy of the surface epithelium of the endolymphatic duct. In addition, some animals showed otospongiotic changes of the bone of the external meatus and otic capsule [34]. Hearing loss and vestibular dysfunction could be found in some of their animals [33]. These studies suggest that autoimmunity to type II collagen may underlie such disorders as otosclerosis, Ménière's disease, and SNHL associated with relapsing polychondritis. Several subsequent studies have both corroborated [35–37] and refuted these findings [38, 39]. We investigated the possible creation of an animal model of autoimmune inner ear dysfunction resulting from exposure to heterologous cochlear tissue [40]. Guinea pigs immunized with fresh bovine cochlear antigen in Freund's adjuvant developed significant hearing loss compared with a control group of animals. In the experimental group, the presence of anticochlear antibodies was uniformly detected and 32% of those ears tested (12 or 38) had significant hearing losses. Histologic evidence of immunologic injury was characterized by spiral ganglion cell degeneration, perivascular infiltration by plasma cells, edema, and hemorrhage. Analysis of their serum by Western blot revealed an antibody that was seen in the animals with hearing loss, but not in those immunized whose hearing was maintained. This suggests that a specific anticochlear autoantibody was responsible for the hearing loss.

In a recent study we extended this observation to patients with progressive SNHL and found that 19 of 54 patients (35%) showed evidence of a specific anticochlear antibody in their serum [41]. Of note, the inner ear antigenic epitope, against which their serum reacted, was the same by molecular weight determination (62,000–68,000) as was found in the experimental autoimmune SNHL produced in guinea pigs. Furthermore, by two-dimensional gel electrophoresis we were able to show that a patient with autoimmune SNHL had autoantibodies that reacted against an inner ear antigen, not only with the same molecular weight as the experimental autoimmune SNHL animals did, but also with the same isoelectric point. This is compelling evidence that some patients with rapidly progressive SNHL have autoantibodies to a particular antigenic epitope within the inner ear and that this is a true organ-specific autoimmune event. This observation has been confirmed by Moscicki [42] in 11 patients, who not only showed the same autoantibody by Western blot analysis, but also showed improved hearing when these patients were given immunosuppressive therapy.

The development of a widely available diagnostic test for this condition awaits further sequencing and synthesis of this specific inner ear antigenic epitope.

References

1   McCabe BF: Autoimmune sensorineural hearing loss. Ann Otol Rhinol Laryngol 1979;88:585.
2   Gussen R: Polyarteritis nodosa and deafness: a human temporal bone study. Arch Otorhinolaryngol 1977;217:263.
3   Jenkins HA, Pollak AM, Fisch U: Polyarteritis nodosa as a cause of sudden deafness: a human temporal bone study. Am J Otolaryngol 1981;2:99.
4   Yanagita N, et al: Acute bilateral deafness with nephritis: a human temporal bone study. Laryngoscope 1987;97:345.
5   Alford BR, et al: Physiologic and histopathologic effects of microembolism of the internal auditory artery. Ann Otol Rhinol Laryngol 1965;74:738.

6   Kimura R, Perlman HB: Arterial obstruction of the labyrinth: I. Cochlear changes;
     II. Vestibular changes. Ann Otol Rhinol Laryngol 1958;67:5.
7   Cody DT, Sones DA: Relapsing polychondritis: audiovestibular manifestations.
     Laryngoscope 1971;81:1208.
8   Cogan DG: Syndrome of nonsyphilitic interstitial keratitis and vestibuloauditory
     symptoms. Arch Ophthalmol 1945;33:144.
9   Haynes BF, et al: Cogan's syndrome: studies in thirteen patients, long-term follow-
     up, and a review of the literature. Medicine 1980;56:426.
10   Fisher ER, Hellstrom HR: Cogan's syndrome and systemic vascular disease. Arch
     Pathol 1961;72:96.
11   Wolff D, et al: The pathology of Cogan's syndrome causing profound deafness. Ann
     Otol Rhinol Laryngol 1965;74:507.
12   Zechner G: Zum Cogan-Syndrom. Acta Otolaryngol (Stockh) 1980;89:310.
13   Rarey KE, Bicknell JM, Davis LE: Labyrinthine osteogenesis in Cogan's syndrome.
     Am J Otolaryngol 1986;4:387.
14   Schuknecht HF: Presentation; Collegium ORLAS, Basel, Switzerland, August 19–
     22, 1990.
15   Paterson PY: Autoimmune neurological disease: experimental animal systems and
     implications for multiple sclerosis; in Talal N (ed): Autoimmunity: Genetic, Immu-
     nologic, Virologic, and Clinical Aspects. New York, Academic Press, 1977.
16   Harris JP: Immunology of the inner ear: response of the inner ear to antigen chal-
     lenge. Otolaryngol Head Neck Surg 1983;91:17.
17   Mogi G, Lim D, Watanabe N: Immunologic study on the inner ear. Arch Otol 1982;
     108:270.
18   Palva T, Raunio V: Disc electrophoretic studies of human perilymph. Ann Otol
     Rhinol Laryngol 1981;76:23.
19   Arnold W, Altermatt HJ, Gebbers JO: Demonstration of immunoglobulins (SIgA,
     IgG) in the human endolymphatic sac. Laryngol Rhinol Otol 1984;63:464.
20   Harris JP: Immunology of the inner ear: evidence of local antibody production. Ann
     Otol Rhinol Laryngol 1984;93:157.
21   Harris JP, Fukuda S, Keithley EM: Spiral modiolar vein: its importance in inner ear
     inflammation. Acta Otolaryngol (Stockh); in press.
22   Gloddek B, Harris JP: Role of lymphokines in the immune response of the inner ear.
     Acta Otolaryngol (Stockh) 1989;108:68–75.
23   Lim D, Silver P: The endolymphatic duct system: a light and electron microscopic
     investigation; in Pulec J (ed): Proceedings of Barany Society Meeting, Los Angeles,
     Calif. 1974.
24   Rask-Anderson H, Stahle J: Immunodefense of the inner ear? Acta Otolaryngol
     (Stockh) 1980;89:283.
25   Takahashi M, Harris JP: Analysis of immunocompetent cells following inner ear
     immunostimulation. Laryngoscope 1988;98:1133–1138.
26   Takahashi M, Harris JP: Anatomic distribution and localization of immunocompe-
     tent cells in normal mouse endolymphatic sac. Acta Otolaryngol (Stockh) 1988;106:
     409–416.
27   Tomiyama S, Harris JP: The role of the endolymphatic sac in inner ear immunity.
     Acta Otolaryngol (Stockh) 1987;103:182.

28 Tomiyama S, Harris JP: Elevation of inner ear antibody levels following direct antigen challenge of the endolymphatic sac. Acta Otolaryngol (Stockh) 1989;107: 202–209.

29 Tomiyama S, Harris JP: Alteration of inner ear responses by endolymphatic duct obstruction. Ann Otol Rhinol Laryngol; in press.

30 Morgenstern C, Ikeda M, Ninoyu O, Koldovsky P: The role of endolymphatic sac in immune response of the inner ear; in Veldman JE (ed): Immunobiology, Histophysiology, Tumor Immunology in Otorhinolaryngology. Amsterdam/Berkeley, Kugler Publications, 1987, pp 131–139.

31 Beickert P: Zur Frage der Empfindungsschwerhörigkeit und Autoallergie. Z Laryngol Rhinol Otol 1961;54:837.

32 Terayama Y, Saski Y: Studies on experimental allergic (isoimmune) labyrinthitis in guinea pigs. Acta Otolaryngol (Stockh) 1963;58:49.

33 Yoo TJ, et al: Type II collagen-induced autoimmune sensorineural hearing loss and vestibular dysfunction in rats. Ann Otol Rhinol Laryngol 1983;92:267.

34 Yoo TJ, et al: Type II collagen-induced autoimmune otospongiosis: a preliminary report. Ann Otol Rhinol Laryngol 1983;92:103.

35 Ohashi T, Tomoda K, Yoshie N: Electrocochleographic changes in endolymphatic hydrops induced by type II collagen immunization through the stylomastoid foramen. Ann Otol Rhinol Laryngol 1989;98:556–562.

36 Huang CC, Yi ZX, Abramson M: Type II collagen-induced otospongiosis-like lesions in rats. Am J Otolaryngol 1986;7:258–266.

37 Soliman AM: Type II collagen-induced inner ear disease: critical evaluation of the guinea pig model. Am J Otol 1990;11:27–32.

38 Harris JP, Woolf NK, Ryan AF: A reexamination of experimental type II collagen autoimmunity: middle and inner ear morphology and function. Ann Otol Rhinol Laryngol 1986;95:176–180.

39 Slvsten-Srensen M, Nielsen LP, Bretlau P, Jorgensen MD: The role of type II collagen autoimmunity in otosclerosis revisited. Acta Otolaryngol (Stockh) 1988;105: 242–247.

40 Harris JP: Experimental autoimmune sensorineural hearing loss. Laryngoscope 1987;97:63–76.

41 Harris JP, Sharp P: Inner ear autoantibodies in patients with rapidly progressive sensorineural hearing loss. Laryngoscope 1990;100:516–524.

42 Moscicki R: Western blot analysis of serum antibody to inner ear antigens in patients with idiopathic progressive bilateral sensorineural hearing loss (IPBSNHL). American Neurotology Society Meeting, Palm Beach, Fla, April 27–29, 1990.

Jeffrey P. Harris, MD, PhD, Division of Otolaryngology-Head and Neck Surgery, University of California, San Diego Medical Center, 225 Dickinson Street, H-895, San Diego, CA 92103 (USA)

Pfaltz CR, Arnold W, Kleinsasser O (eds): Bearing of Basic Research on Clinical Otolaryngology. Adv Otorhinolaryngol. Basel, Karger, 1991, vol 46, pp 34–49

Vimentin as a Possible Cytoskeletal Marker for Regeneration in the Human Cochlea[1]

Matti Anniko[a], *Wolfgang Arnold*[b]
in cooperation with Lars-Eric Thornell[c], *Frans C.S. Ramaekers*[d], *Ismo Virtanen*[e]

Departments of Oto-Rhino-Laryngology and Head & Neck Surgery,
[a] University Hospital, Uppsala, Sweden; [b] Kantonsspital, Luzern, Switzerland;
[c] Department of Anatomy, University of Umeå, Sweden;
[d] Department of Pathology, University of Nijmegen, The Netherlands;
[e] Department of Anatomy, University of Helsinki, Finland

Lethal damage to the highly specialized epithelial cell types of the membranous labyrinth in the inner ear of higher vertebrates, in particular the hair cells (HCs), has so far been considered as irreversible. There are a number of inner ear diseases that can exert a reversible effect on hearing, but have different pathophysiological mechanisms. Clinically reversible changes in cochlear function can be detected, for instance in certain immunologically mediated dysfunctions of hearing when treated with steroids (the stria vascularis (SV) as the primary target?). In Alport's syndrome, recovery of hearing loss has been described following renal transplantation and therapy with immunosuppressive drugs [1–4]. Although permanent deafness can ensue following the administration of the ototoxic loop diuretic furosemide or ethacrynic acid (the SV as the primary target), hearing in most cases returns to pretreatment values when administration of the drug is stopped, provided that it has been given in clinically adequate doses (following both single and repeated injections) [5]. Even in patients treated with aminoglycoside antibiotics (the HCs as the primary target)

[1] This study was supported by grants from the Swedish Medical Research Council (12X-7305), the Ragnar and Torsten Söderberg Foundation, the Foundation Tysta Skolan and the Swiss National Research Council (32-26319.89).

and as an adverse effect causing hearing impairment, some reversibility may be found after a lapse of time [6].

In Ménière's disease, mechanical damage to the epithelial lining of scala media has been regarded as one possible pathophysiological mechanism, for instance rupture of Reissner's membrane or changes in the ionic fluxes through tight junctions or membranes at the level of the organ of Corti [7, 8]. At least at the early stages this disease is self-limiting, and has periods of regeneration of hearing.

For obvious reasons it is not known how far the morphological changes can progress in the human at the cellular and subcellular levels before the possibility of regeneration of function is irrevocably lost.

In avians, degenerated HCs can be replaced by regeneration – at least following ototoxic drug insult [9] and acoustic trauma [10, 11]. In amphibians and some fishes, auditory sensory HCs are produced throughout life as well as in response to injury [12]. In both mammals and birds, however, the production of cochlear HCs is thought to cease after early embryogenesis [13, 14]. Embryonically, HC addition occurs along the edges of the growing epithelium [15, 16]. However, proliferation occurs throughout the sensory region of the crista ampullaris and possibly other end organs during later stages of development in the mouse [16]. Posttrauma HC replacement in birds occurs at the site of damage [10, 11].

Lethal cellular damage requires morphologic regeneration in order to re-establish highly specialized function. Several earlier detailed consecutive experimental studies have analyzed the incorporation of thymidine as a marker for regeneration in the inner ear [17, 18]. For obvious reasons this is not possible when analyzing the human labyrinth.

In a series of recent papers we have described the complexity of the cytoskeleton of inner ear cells as shown by the expression of intermediate filaments (IFs), particularly the pattern of cytokeratins [19–21]. In the present study the distribution of vimentin (a subgroup of IFs) is analyzed in the fetal and adult human cochlea with reference to vimentin as a cytoskeletal marker of mesenchymal cells or cells with a potentially mesenchymal-like cytoskeleton and thus likely to constitute a morphological basis for regenerative properties.

Material and Methods

The entire material comprises sections stained for vimentin, taken from 8 fetal (9–20 gestational weeks (GW)) and 4 adult (38–69 years old) human temporal bones.

Each temporal bone was sectioned serially (4 μm thick). Fetal temporal bones with an age of 9–16 GW were initially shock-frozen in isopentane cooled with liquid nitrogen slush and cryosectioned (at −40 °C) whereas 18–20 GW inner ears were initially lightly fixed in paraformaldehyde prior to cryosectioning. The adult temporal bones were initially fixed in sublimate-formaldehyde and decalcified in EDTA prior to sectioning. A detailed analysis of different technical procedures for preservation of antigenicity in the fetal and adult human inner ear for immunomorphology, using a large number of well-characterized monoclonal antibodies (mAbs), has been published recently [22]. All sections comprised the cochlea but in many the vestibular part of the labyrinth had also been included. When possible, appropriate comparisons are made vis-à-vis the vestibular organs.

Every tenth section was stained with hematoxylin and eosin to facilitate orientation. Based on these findings, appropriate sections were taken for incubation with mAbs for vimentin. The following well-characterized mAbs were used: RV 202, RV 203, K-17, vimentin Bio-Genex®, vimentin 3B4 and vimentin-24 [22]. The peroxidase-antiperoxidase (PAP) technique was used for staining. The sections were analyzed and photographed in a Zeiss Axiophot light microscope. Each section was also viewed in phase contrast to further enhance orientation.

Results

In the *fetal* cochlea, positivity for vimentin (with all mAbs) was found in all epithelial cells of the receding greater epithelial ridge (GER) but with particularly strong expression in the most apical cell cytoplasm of the uppermost cell layer, i.e. the area for secretion of organic material to form the tectorial membrane (fig. 1, 3, 4). The epithelial cells of the spiral limbus showed immunoreactivity with increasing positivity towards the cell surface, i.e. where the tectorial membrane inserts. The marginal cells of the SV were stained when using incubation with mAbs RV 202 but not when using the other five mAbs. This difference was verified in consecutive sections from different temporal bones.The other cell layers of the SV stained for vimentin, showing differentiation into intermediate and basal cells. Otherwise the staining pattern in the cochleae was the same using all six different mAbs.

All mesenchymal cells, including the mesenchymal layer of Reissner's membrane, expressed vimentin. In comparison, all supporting cells in the maculae and cristae stained for vimentin – but not the HCs. Positivity occurred for all mesenchymal cells (fig. 2).

In the *adult* normal cochlea the staining for vimentin in the epithelial layer was restricted to only few but distinct cell types – the inner and outer

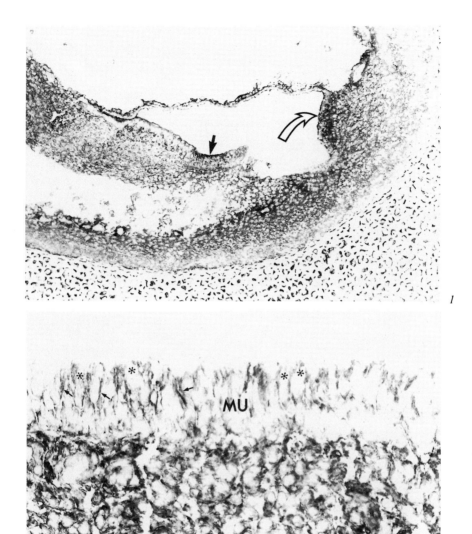

Fig. 1. Human cochlea at 14th GW. Section immunostained for vimentin using mAbs RV 202. Positivity is evident not only in all mesenchymal cells but also in areas of the epithelial lining of the scala media: the receding GER (unfilled arrow) and the future marginal cells (filled arrow) in the SV.

Fig. 2. The same temporal bone as in figure 1, showing a section through the macula utriculi (MU) immunostained with mAbs RV 202. Staining is obvious in mesenchymal cells and the supporting cells (arrows) between the individual HCs (asterisks) which do not stain.

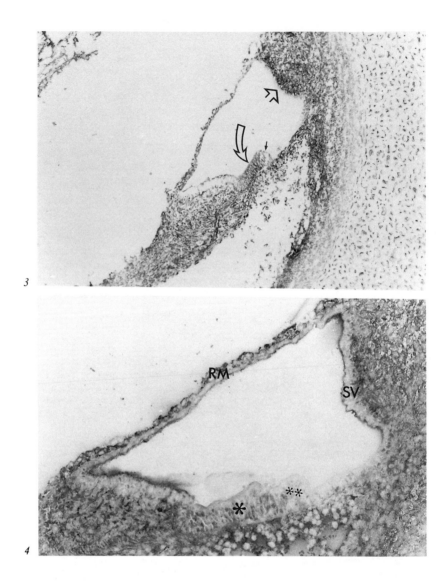

Fig. 3. Human cochlea at GW 14. Section immunostained for vimentin, using mAbs RV 203. Mesenchymal cells show positivity, whereas in the epithelial lining of the scala media, staining occurs only in the receding GER (curved unfilled arrow) but not in the epithelium of the lesser epithelial ridge (filled arrow) or in the dark cell area (open arrow) of the future SV.

Fig. 4. Human cochlea, GW 16. Section immunostained for vimentin, using mAbs K-17. Positivity is obvious in all mesenchymal cells and to some extent in the GER (large asterisk) but not in the lesser epithelial ridge (double small asterisks) or in marginal cells of SV. At the insertion of the tectorial membrane in the spiral limbus area, some staining occurs which is not present in control experiments. RM = Reissner's membrane.

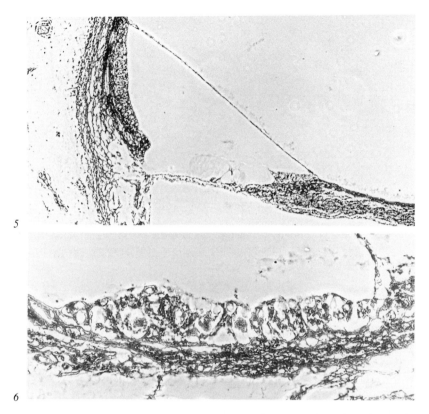

Fig. 5. Adult human cochlea. Section immunostained for vimentin, using mAbs from Bio-Genex®. Positivity occurs in all mesenchymal cells but also in inner and outer pillar cells in the organ of Corti and some cells in the epithelial lining of the SV.

Fig. 6. Detail from the SV of the cochlea shown in figure 5. Positivity is evident not only in the supporting cells in the spiral ligament but also in basal, intermediate and some (marginal?) cells adjacent to the surface of the SV.

pillar cells, some cells in the spiral limbus and root cells close to the spiral prominence (fig. 5, 8, 12). The latter also stained strongly for vasoactive intestinal polypeptide (VIP) (fig. 13) [Anniko and Arnold, unpubl. data, 1990]. Immunoreactivity for vimentin occurred in intermediate and basal cells of the SV (fig. 6) and all mesenchymal cells including the Schwann cells surrounding the nerve fibers and spiral ganglion cells (fig. 7, 9). A

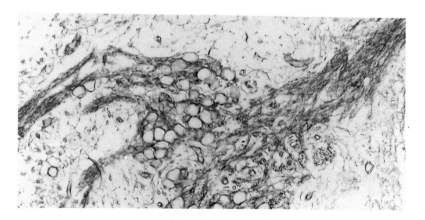

Fig. 7. Spiral ganglion from an adult human cochlea immunostained for vimentin with mAbs from Bio-Genex®. Positivity is evident in mesenchymal cells and the Schwann cells surrounding spiral ganglion cells.

certain variation in the extent of staining was correlated to the individual mAbs, but not regarding the staining pattern.

In vestibular organs, staining for vimentin followed the same pattern as for fetal organs – positivity in all mesenchymal cells, for instance the cells forming the trabecular network in the perilymphatic space but also in groups of cells in the epithelial lining of semicircular canals (fig. 11). Using our mAbs, positivity for vimentin was weak in supporting epithelial cells adjacent to vestibular HCs, irrespective of any of the five vestibular end organs (fig. 10).

In adult cochleae with varying degrees of degeneration of the organ of Corti, the staining for vimentin was just as scarce as during normal conditions. However, additional positivity was identified in inner border cells and in groups of outer sulcus cells (fig. 14).

In the partially degenerated adult SV a few cells lining the endolymphatic space displayed positivity for vimentin (fig. 15). Our interpretation was that the degeneration was rather inactive, showing morphologically a partially atrophic SV with blood vessels surrounded by intensely staining cells. In contrast, sections from the adult SV of the Shaker-2 mouse prior to obvious morphologic degeneration showed an intense coexpression of both vimentin and cytokeratins in all three cell layers (fig.16–18) [Anniko and Arnold, unpubl. data, 1990].

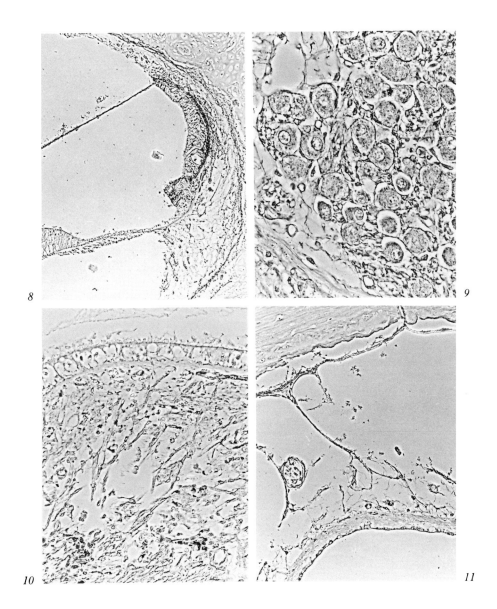

Fig. 8, 9. Adult human cochlea. Sections immunostained for vimentin with mAbs 3B4. Positivity is particularly intense below the basal cells in the spiral ligament and in some cells (root cells?) in the spiral prominence (fig. 8). In the spiral ganglion, staining is evident both in spiral ganglion cells and in surrounding Schwann cells (fig. 9).

Fig. 10, 11. Adult human inner ear. Sections immunostained for vimentin with mAbs 3B4. Staining is evident in mesenchymal cells in the crista ampullaris (fig. 10) and in the interconnecting cells in the perilymphatic space of the semicircular canals and in some epithelial cells lining the endolymphatic space (fig. 11).

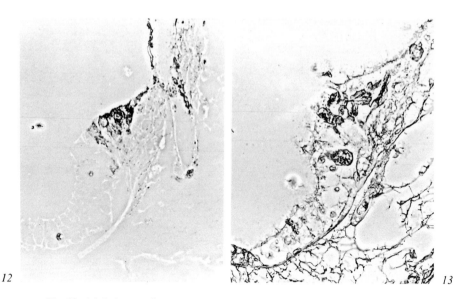

12
13

Fig. 12. Adult human inner ear. Section through the cochlea, showing the spiral prominence and adjacent cells. Immunostaining for vimentin with mAbs from Bio-Genex®. Intense positivity in a few cells close to the SV.

Fig. 13. A rather adjacent serial section to that in figure 12 immunostained with mAbs identifying VIP. Intense staining occurs in the same cells as those immunostained for vimentin in figure 12.

Discussion

The mammalian cytoskeleton is a highly integrated structural network comprising three major classes of filamentous polymers: microfilaments, microtubules and IFs. Changes in cell shape and motility are the result of directed alterations of cytoskeletal dynamics: filaments polymerize, depolymerize, contract, elongate, and change their position. The cytoskeleton is integrally involved in a variety of cell functions, including force production and transduction, cell surface modulation, phagocytosis, secretion, intracellular transport, organelle translocation, cell migration, and mitogenesis [23].

IFs (10 nm in diameter) are midway in size between microfilaments and microtubules. Five types of IF proteins exist – vimentin, cytokeratins, desmin, neurofilament triplet proteins and glial fibrillary acidic protein [24]. Each specific cell type exhibits its own characteristic pattern of

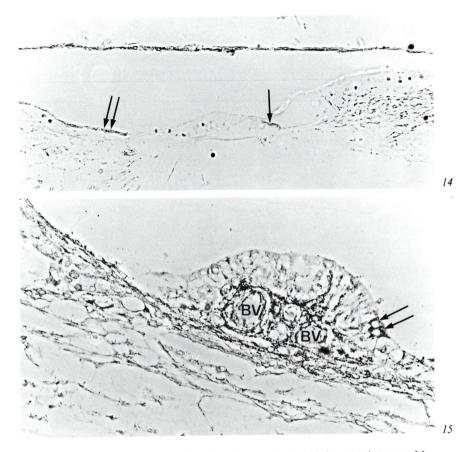

14

15

Fig. 14, 15. Adult human cochlea, showing morphological degeneration caused by repeated treatment with cisplatin because of a head and neck carcinoma. Immunostaining for vimentin using mAbs from Bio-Genex®. Positivity occurs in epithelial cells in the outer sulcus area (double arrows), the inner border cell (arrow) and in epithelial cells of Reissner's membrane (fig. 14). In the SV (fig. 15), there is positivity around blood vessels (BV) and in several cells (arrows) reaching the endolymphatic surface.

expression. At the ultrastructural level all IFs show the same morphological features and it is not possible to identify any of the subclasses. In addition, ordinary fixation procedures for electron microscopy destroy the cytoskeletal network of IFs. There is a continuous pattern of IFs from the nucleus of one cell to its neighbor via points of cell-cell and cell-substratum contact [25]. Recently, distinct sites for attachment of vimentin to both the

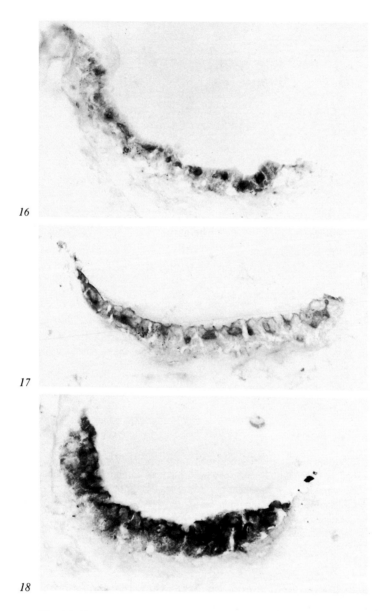

16

17

18

Fig. 16–18. Adult (2-month-old) inner ear of the Shaker-2 mouse mutant. Sections through the SV immunostained for vimentin (mAbs vimentin-24; fig. 16), cytokeratin No. 18 (mAbs RPN 1160; fig. 17) and cytokeratin No. 8 (mAbs RPN 1164; fig. 18). Coexpression of vimentin and cytokeratins is evident in at least marginal and intermediate cells.

nuclear envelope and the plasma membrane have been identified [26]. For this reason, IFs are commonly regarded as spatial integrators [27]. The expression o various types of IFs is cell type specific and is related to pathways of embryonic differentiation [28].

We have recently demonstrated a specific pattern of cytokeratin networks in the adult human cochlea and vestibular organs, hypothesizing their functional significance as providing a pancellular type of rigidity both in the organ of Corti (with gradients both within the organ of Corti at the same level and with a base to apex directed gradient of increasing stiffness) and in the vestibular sense organs [20, 21, 29]. In such a way these proteins could influence both the macro- and micromechanics in the perception of the travelling wave (hearing) respectively during movement of endolymph at spatial movements (balance). Thus, the assumed role of IFs in maintaining the shape and rigidity of individual cells may be of particular significance in the organ of Corti and the vestibular neurosensory epithelium, where the transduction of pressure waves to electrical impulses is regulated largely by the mechanical properties of sensory and supporting cells.

Analyses on the distribution of vimentin in the adult mammalian inner ear have been reported previously but only in the gerbil [30]. Positivity was found in Deiters' cells, inner phalangeal cells, Böttcher's cells, some outer sulcus cells, and in the basal and intermediate cells of the SV. In the vestibular system, type I HCs showed intense immunostaining for vimentin, whereas the adjacent supporting epithelia stained considerably less. A slightly different pattern was found in our study of the fetal and adult human labyrinth. In the adult human, all HCs lack expression of any of the five subclasses of IFs, whereas in the fetal cochlea, immunoreactivity for vimentin has been demonstrated in fetal outer HCs with a gradient of decreasing positivity from the first to the third row at the same level in the cochlea [31].

Species differences and differences in the specificity of mAbs as well as differences in technical methods may account for some of the discrepancies between adult cochleae from the two species. With regard to previous extensive systematic analyses of techniques for immunomorphology of the fetal and adult human labyrinth, we consider our technique in the present study to be the optimal one [22].

The expression of vimentin in human epithelial cells of the membranous labyrinth was seen to change with increasing differentiation of the inner ear. In the adult normal cochlea, positivity for vimentin was localized distinctly to only a few morphologically well-defined epithelial cell types – inner and outer pillar cells and epithelial cells at the spiral limbus and the spiral prominence (root cells). In contrast, in sections where varying degrees of pathology were found in the organ of Corti and the SV, positivity for vimentin was also identified in some outer sulcus cells and the epithelial lining towards the spiral prominence.

All mammalian HCs have a principally similar morphology but species differences do occur, for instance between the human and a number of rodent species which are often used in experimental studies on the inner ear [32]. Regeneration of HCs has so far not been described in higher vertebrates, but does occur in some amphibians and birds. In the adult human cochlea particularly, inner HCs are found with giant sensory hairs. This morphologically specific feature has been interpreted both as regeneration of the highly specialized suprastructures of individual HCs following sublethal damage and as a way to protect the HCs from extensive mechanical shearing by the travelling wave by raising the overlying tectorial membrane. In the adult Coturnix quail the potential for HC regeneration after trauma appears to be age-related, indicating that there may be a critical period during which recovery is possible [11]. Although vimentin (coexpressed with cytokeratins) is identified in fetal human outer HCs, the IF type of cytoarchitecture is lost during the final cytodifferentiation of HCs, i.e. the cytoskeleton changes prior to the onset of HC function [19, 31]. Recently, Girod et al. [33] analyzed possible precursors for regenerating HCs in the avian cochlea following acoustic trauma. It was hypothesized that cuboidal epithelial cells lateral to the sensory region (similar to the outer sulcus cells in the human) may serve as a latent stem cell population. In our study we found expression of vimentin in outer sulcus cells in specimens where the organ of Corti had been damaged. An expression of vimentin may precede a cell's commitment to terminal differentiation [34]. It is thus tempting to speculate that a change in the expression of IF type indicates some type of regenerative focus, i.e. having the potential to activate a latent production of vimentin into the cell cytoskeleton.

It is well known that, on exposure to a changed microenvironment, epithelial cells can switch to another type of gene-regulated production of cytoskeletal proteins. For instance, Madin-Darby kidney cells cultured under conditions that allow extensive cell-cell contact synthesize much cytokeratin and little vimentin, but when cell-cell contact is limited, these cells express abundant vimentin and very low levels of cytokeratins [35]. Although epithelial cells grown in culture under certain conditions can express vimentin-type IFs, this is an unusual property for epithelial cells in vivo under normal conditions.

Trauma leading to morphological changes modulates the internal relationships of adjacent cells and may induce changes in the formation of cytoskeletal proteins. In the Shaker-2 mouse a slowly progressing degeneration of the SV occurs during the first months of life [36]. This mutant never attains a normal electrophysiological function before the hereditary-induced degeneration starts. For this reason, immunomorphological analyses of biochemically or morphologically completely normal SV cannot be made [37]. However, expression of vimentin does occur in these marginal cells, irrespective of age, but not in marginal cells of the adult normal mouse [Anniko and Arnold, unpubl. data, 1990]. Also in this part of the cochlea, an expression of vimentin is found in cells undergoing morphological changes (rebuilding of the cytoskeleton), but not in corresponding cells under normal conditions.

To summarize, the location of epithelial cells with expression of vimentin in the adult human cochlea coincides with hypothesized stem cell areas having regenerative potential in the cochlea of lower vertebrates. Vimentin can constitute a cytoskeletal marker for regenerative foci.

References

1 McDonald T, Zincke H, Anderson C, Ott N: Reversal of deafness after renal transplantation in Alport's syndrome. Laryngoscope 1978;88:38–42.
2 Arnold W: Ototoxizität durch Schleifendiuretika. Münch Med Wochenschr 1982; 124:271–274.
3 Mitschke H, Schmidt P, Zazgornik J, Kopsa H, Puls P: Effect of renal transplantation on uremic deafness, a long-term study. Audiology 1977;16:530–534.
4 Arnold W: Inner ear and renal diseases. Ann Otol Rhinol Laryngol 1984;93(suppl 112):119–123.
5 Anniko M: Principles in cochlear toxicity. Arch Toxicol 1985(suppl 8):218–237.
6 Rybak LP: Ototoxic mechanisms; in Altschuler RA, Hoffman DW, Bobbin RP (eds): Neurobiology of Hearing: The Cochlea. New York, Raven Press, 1986, pp 441–454.
7 Nadol JB (ed): Ménière's Disease. Amsterdam, Kugler & Ghedini, 1989.
8 Jahnke K: Diagnosis and treatment of disorders of vestibular system: electron microscopic investigations and pathophysiological aspects; in New Dimensions in Otorhinolaryngology – Head and Neck Surgery. New York, Elsevier Science, 1985, pp 135–140.
9 Cruz MR, Lambert PR, Rubel EW: Light microscopic evidence of hair cell regeneration after gentamicin toxicity in chick cochlea. Arch Otolaryngol Head Neck Surg 1987;113:1058–1062.

10   Corwin JT, Cotanche DA: Regeneration of sensory cells after acoustic trauma. Science 1988;240:1772–1774.

11   Ryals BM, Rubel EW: Hair cell regeneration after acoustic trauma in adult Coturnix quail. Science 1988;240:1774–1776.

12   Corwin JT: Perpetual production of hair cells and maturational changes in hair cell ultrastructure accompany postembryonic growth in an amphibian ear. Proc Natl Acad Sci USA 1985;82:3911–3915.

13   Ruben RJ: Development of the inner ear of the mouse: a radioautographic study of terminal mitoses. Acta Otolaryngol (Stockh) 1967(suppl 220):1–44.

14   Rubel EW: Ontogeny of structure and function in the vertebrate auditory system; in Jacobson M (ed): Handbook of Sensory Physiology, vol 9: Development of Sensory Systems. New York, Springer, 1978.

15   Li CW: Hair cell development in the inner ear. Scan Electron Microsc 1978;2:967–974.

16   Lim DJ, Anniko M: Developmental morphology of the inner ear: a scanning electron microscopic observation. Acta Otolaryngol (Stockh) 1985(suppl 442):1–69.

17   Popper AN, Hoxter B: Growth of the fish ear. II. Location of newly proliferated sensory cells in the saccular epithelium of *Astronotus ocellatus.* Hear Res 1990;45: 33–40.

18   Presson JC, Popper AN: Possible precursors to new hair cells, support cells, and Schwann cells in the ear of a postembryonic fish. Hear Res 1990;46:9–22.

19   Anniko M, Thornell L-E, Ramaekers FCS, Stigbrand T: Cytokeratin diversity in epithelia of the human inner ear. Acta Otolaryngol (Stockh) 1989;108:385–396.

20   Anniko M, Arnold W, Thornell L-E, Virtanen I, Ramaekers FCS: Regional variations in the expression of cytokeratin proteins in the adult human cochlea. Eur Arch Otorhinolaryngol 1990;247:182–188.

21   Arnold W, Anniko M: Das Zytokeratinskelett des menschlichen Corti-Organs und seine funktionelle Bedeutung. Laryngol Rhinol Otol 1990;69:24–30.

22   Anniko M, Arnold W: Methods for cellular and subcellular visualization of intermediate filament proteins in the human inner ear. Acta Otolaryngol (Stockh) 1990 (suppl 470):13–22.

23   Stein W, Bronner F (eds): Cell Shape. Determinants, Regulation and Regulatory Role. New York, Academic Press 1989, pp 1–433.

24   Schliwa M: The cytoskeleton. Wien, Springer, 1986, pp 1–326.

25   Fey EG, Wan KM, Penman S: Epithelial cytoskeletal framework and nuclear matrix-intermediate filament scaffold, three-dimensional organization and protein composition. J Cell Biol 1984;98:1973–1984.

26   Georgatos SD, Blobel G: Two distinct attachment sites for vimentin along the plasma membrane and nuclear envelope in avian erythrocytes: a basis for vectorial assembly of intermediate filaments. J Cell Biol 1987;105:105–115.

27   Lazarides E: Intermediate filaments as mechanical integrators of cellular space. Nature (Lond) 1980;283:249–256.

28   Osborn M, Weber K: Intermediate filament proteins: a multigene family distinguishing major cell lineages. Trends Biochem Sci 1986;11:469–472.

29   Arnold W, Anniko M, Pfaltz CR: Funktionelle Morphologie der äusseren Haarzellen des Menschen: Neue Aspekte. Laryngol Rhinol Otol (Stuttg) 1990;69:177–186.

30 Schulte BA, Adams JC: Immunohistochemical localization of vimentin in the gerbil inner ear. J Histochem Cytochem 1989;37:1787–1797.

31 Anniko M, Thornell L-E, Virtanen I: Cytoskeletal organization of the human inner ear. II. Characterization of intermediate filaments in the cochlea. Acta Otolaryngol (Stockh) 1987(suppl 437):29–54.

32 Arnold W, Anniko M: Structurally based new functional interpretations of the subsurface cisternal network in human outer hair cells. Acta Otolaryngol (Stockh) 1990; 109:213–220.

33 Girod DA, Duckert LG, Rubel EW: Possible precursors of regenerated hair cells in the avian cochlea following acoustic trauma. Hear Res 1989;42:175–194.

34 Ngai J, Capetanaki YG, Lazarides E: Differentiation of murine erythroleukemia cells results in the rapid repression of vimentin gene expression. J Cell Biol 1984;99: 306–314.

35 Ben-Ze'ev A: Cell-cell interaction and cell configuration related control of cytokeratins and vimentin expression in epithelial cells and in fibroblasts. Ann NY Acad Sci 1985;455:597–612.

36 Anniko M: Specific pathology in the stria vascularis in postnatal progressive genetic inner ear disorder. Hear Res 1982;6:247–258.

37 Anniko M, Wróblewski R: Deterioration of the elemental composition of endolymph in genetic inner ear disease. Arch Otorhinolaryngol 1980;228:171–186.

Prof. Matti Anniko, Department of Oto-Rhino-Laryngology and Head & Neck Surgery, University Hospital, S-751 85 Uppsala (Sweden)

Pfaltz CR, Arnold W, Kleinsasser O (eds): Bearing of Basic Research on Clinical Otolaryngology. Adv Otorhinolaryngol. Basel, Karger, 1991, vol 46, pp 50–70

Ear Pathology in Autoimmune Disease[1]

Harold F. Schuknecht

Department of Otology and Laryngology, Harvard Medical School, and
Department of Otolaryngology, Massachusetts Eye and Ear Infirmary,
Boston, Mass., USA

Audiovestibular manifestations are a common occurrence in several systemic (nonorgan-specific) autoimmune diseases but may also present as an organ-specific autoimmune entity. While the external and middle ear can be involved, particularly in relapsing polychondritis and Wegener's granulomatosis where the eustachian tube is blocked, the more devastating autoimmune phenomena involve the inner ear.

The most common nonorgan-specific autoimmune diseases that involve the inner ear are polyarteritis nodosa and Cogan's syndrome. Less commonly, the inner ear may be involved in relapsing polychondritis, Vogt-Koyanagi-Harada syndrome, giant cell arteritis, Takayasu's disease, hypersensitivity vasculitis (small vessel involvement), sarcoidosis, and systemic lupus erythematosus (table 1).

Nonorgan-Specific Autoimmune Disease

Polyarteritis nodosa

Polyarteritis nodosa is a necrotizing vasculitis of small- and medium-sized arteries [1]. Because of the widespread involvement of arteries, the disease can present a myriad of symptoms including malaise, weight loss,

[1] This study was supported by Grant DC 00079 from the National Institutes of Health/National Institute on Deafness and Other Communication Disorders and by a grant from the Deafness Research Foundation, New York, in support of the National Temporal Bone Bank Program.

Table 1. Audiovestibular symptoms

Autoimmune diseases	Temporal bone studies
Polyarteritis nodosa	4 cases
Cogan's syndrome	3 cases
Relapsing polychondritis	1 case
Vogt-Koyanagi-Harada syndrome	
Giant cell arteritis	
Takayasu's disease	
Hypersensitivity vasculitis (small vessel)	
Sarcoidosis	
Systemic lupus erythematosus	

anorexia, fever, arthritis, neuropathy, hypertension, abdominal pain, and renal insufficiency. The diagnosis ultimately depends on the demonstration of necrotizing arteritis by biopsy of involved muscle or other organs.

Sensorineural hearing loss may occur as an initial manifestation prior to the onset of other manifestations of the disease or after the disease has been well established. The hearing loss may be unilateral or bilateral, and the onset is often sudden or rapidly progressive and profound.

Temporal bone studies have been reported on 4 cases of polyarteritis nodosa with audiovestibular symptoms (table 2) [2–5]. Involvement was unilateral in 1 and bilateral in 3. The onset was sudden and profound in 4 ears, sudden and progressive in 2 ears, and sudden and limited to high tones in 1 ear. Vertigo was acute and severe in 1 case, mild in 2, and not mentioned in 1.

There was severe degeneration of the organ of Corti with total loss of hair cells in 6 of the 7 ears (table 3). The ear with the high tone loss had only a basal turn lesion. The vestibular sense organs were severely degenerated in 1 ear, normal in 4, and not mentioned in 2. Endolymphatic hydrops was moderate in 1 ear, mild in 1, absent in 3, and not mentioned in 2. Fibrous tissue and bone proliferation was present throughout the cochlea and vestibular labyrinth in 1 ear, only in the basal turn in 2 ears, and only in the apical regions in 2 ears.

It seems probable that the inner ear pathology is caused by obliterative vasculitis of the labyrinthine artery or its branches resulting in diffuse or focal areas of ischemic necrosis. The inner ear changes therefore do not

Table 2. Autoimmune inner ear disease: temporal bone case reports, clinical manifestations

Case	Author/ref.	Age	Sex	Ear	Duration otol. symptoms	Features of hearing loss	Features of vertigo
Polyarteritis nodosa							
1	Gussen, 1977 [2]	66	F	L	7 months	sudden, profound	not mentioned
2	Jenkins et al., 1981 [3]	48	M	L R	7 months 7 months	sudden, profound sudden, profound	acute, severe, two attacks
3	Yanagita et al., 1987 [4]	37	M	R L	4 months 4 months	sudden, profound sudden, profound	mild
4	Yoon et al., 1989 [5]	54	M	R L	10 months 7 months	sudden, progressive sudden, progressive	mild, occasional
Cogan's syndrome							
5	Fisher and Hellstrom, 1961 [7]	32	M	R L	6 months 6 months	progressive, profound progressive, profound	vertigo was present, presumably mild
6	Wolff et al., 1965 [8]	50	M	R L	11 years 11 years	progressive, profound progressive, profound	moderate, walked with wide base
7	Rarey et al., 1986 [9]	64	M	R L	29 years 29 years	sudden, profound sudden, profound	acute, severe
Relapsing polychondritis							
8	Hoshino et al., 1978 [11], 1980 [12]	56	F	R L	11 months 11 months	sudden, profound sudden, profound	mild, continued unsteadiness

Table 3. Autoimmune inner ear disease: temporal bone case reports, pathological findings

Case	Ear	Degeneration		Endo-lymphatic hydrops	Fibro-osseous reaction
		cochlea	vestibular labyrinth		
Polyarteritis nodosa					
1	L	+++	+++	moderate	cochlea and vestibular labyrinth
2	L	+++	normal	mild	basal turn
	R	+	normal	none	none
3	R	+++	normal	none	apex only
	L	+++	normal	none	apex only
4	R	+++	not stated	not stated	basal turn
	L	+++	not stated	not stated	none
Cogan's syndrome					
5	R	+++	+++	mild	cochlea
	L	+++	+++	mild	cochlea
6	R	+++	+++	severe	cochlea and vestibular labyrinth
	R	+++	+++	severe	cochlea and vestibular labyrinth
7	R	+++	+++	not stated	cochlea and vestibular labyrinth
	L	+++	+++	not stated	cochlea and vestibular labyrinth
Relapsing polychondritis					
8	R	+++	++	none	basal turn and lateral canal
	L	+++	++	none	none

represent autoimmune disease in the sense that the immune system is reacting to proteins of the membranous labyrinth.

The following observations further support an ischemic pathogenesis rather than an inner ear autoimmune reaction in these cases: (1) The clinical features of suddenness of onset and profoundness of hearing loss are consistent with acute obstruction of the labyrinthine artery or the common cochlear artery. (2) The clinical feature of unilateral involvement as occurred in 1 ear cannot be attributed logically to an inner ear autoimmune phenomenon. (3) The demonstration of occluded arteries in the internal auditory canals of case 1 [2] and case 4 [5] support a vascular pathogenesis. (4) The finding of fibrous tissue and bone limited to the apical regions of the cochleas as occurred in case 3 [4] also points toward a vascular pathogenesis for it has been demonstrated experimentally in animals that obstruction of the labyrinthine artery occasionally leads to ischemic degenerative lesions that are most severe in the apex of the cochlea [6].

Case 1 in table 2, reported by Gussen [2]. At age 63 this woman developed an illness which was characterized by weakness and numbness of the extremities, loss of position sense, muscle and joint pain, paresthesias, ankle swelling, and exertional dyspnea. Muscle biopsy revealed an inflammatory myopathy with scattered degenerating and regenerating fibers and focal perivascular collections of lymphocytes and plasma cells. Biopsy of the sural nerve revealed perineural fibrosis and numerous perivascular foci of lymphocytes and plasma cells. The patient was treated at various times with prednisone, Lasix, digoxin, and other medications. She had repeated remissions and relapses and gradual deterioration of health from hypertension, cardiac and renal failure, progressive weakness, and decreasing sensorium. The first notation regarding hearing was 7 months before death when it was noted that there was decreased hearing on the left and normal hearing on the right. No audiometric tests were done. She died at the age of 66. Both clinical and autopsy diagnoses were polyarteritis nodosa.

Histopathology: The cochlea of the left ear shows degeneration of the membranous labyrinth, fibrosis and new bone formation, and endolymphatic hydrops (fig. 1). There is total absence of the organ of Corti, stria vascularis, nerve fibers, and cochlear neurons. The tectorial membrane where evident is fragmented and encapsulated. Fibroareolar tissue and acellular trabecular bone is present in the scala tympani of the hook region. In the middle cochlear turn fibro-osseous tissue fills the scala tympani and is continuous with similar tissue within the scala media through a degenerated basilar membrane. The vestibular system demonstrates extensive fibrosis and bone formation within both perilymphatic and endolymphatic spaces of the semicircular canals and ampullas. There is necrosis of the membranous labyrinth including the utricular and saccular maculas. The cochlear and vestibular nerves are markedly atrophic.

The labyrinthine artery is seen at the meatus of the internal auditory canal (fig. 2). All layers of the arterial wall are thickened. The outer portion of the media shows a thickening by amorphous material in which sparsely occurring smooth muscle cells are seen. The adventitia is thickened with similar amorphous reddish-staining material. The intimal layer is thickened with only a tiny lumen remaining. There is complete degeneration and loss of the internal elastic membrane. No acute or chronic inflamma-

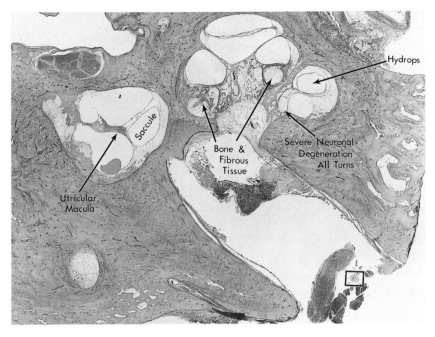

Fig. 1. Polyarteritis nodosa with audiovestibular involvement. Overview of the left temporal bone showing extensive degeneration of the membranous labyrinth, endolymphatic hydrops, and bone and fibrous tissue in the cochlea and vestibular labyrinth. Courtesy of Gussen. See figure 2.

tory cells are seen in the vessel wall. The subarcuate artery as well as arteries at the fundus of the internal auditory canal and in the modiolus show open lumens filled with blood. None appear to be associated with inflammatory cells.

The opposite right ear shows some loss of hair cells and spiral ganglion cells in the basal turn, but otherwise appears normal.

Cogan's Syndrome

Cogan's syndrome, as originally described, consists of nonsyphilitic interstitial keratitis with audiovestibular symptoms, occasionally associated with iritis and subconjunctival hemorrhages. Atypically the patients may develop scleritis, retinal artery occlusion, retinal hemorrhages, papilledema, exophthalmos, and tenonitis, with or without interstitial keratitis. About 70% of the patients have systemic manifestations which include

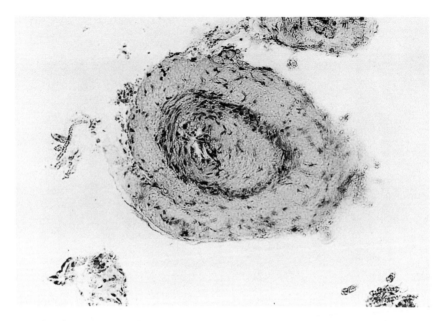

Fig. 2. Framed area in figure 1 showing complete obliteration of the lumen of the labyrinthine (internal auditory) artery. Courtesy of Gussen.

adenopathy, gastrointestinal hemorrhage, aortic regurgitations, musculoskeletal complaints, splenomegaly, and neurologic symptoms. Systemic vasculitis has been found in some patients but it has never been described in the eye or inner ear. The episodes of audiovestibular disorder may occur before or soon after the onset of eye symptoms and consist of unilateral or bilateral sensorineural hearing loss and attacks of severe vertigo with nausea and vomiting which simulate the symptoms of Ménière's disease. If untreated, the hearing loss may rapidly become profound (1–6 months) and irreversible.

The literature reveals 3 temporal bone case reports of patients with Cogan's syndrome (table 2) [7–9]. (A fourth case that was reported as Cogan's syndrome is not included because the patient had a hearing loss in early childhood and there is no record of eye disease or other manifestations of Cogan's syndrome.) All 3 authentic cases had bilateral hearing losses. In 2 cases the hearing losses progressed rapidly to profound deafness and in 1 case the losses were sudden and profound. All 3 had vestibular symptoms.

All 6 cochleas showed diffuse severe degeneration of the organs of Corti and vestibular sense organs with total loss of hair cells (table 3). Endolymphatic hydrops was mild in both ears of 1 case, severe in both ears of 1 case, and not determined because of severe degeneration in both labyrinths in 1 case. Fibrous tissue and bone proliferation involved both the cochleas and vestibular labyrinths in both ears of 2 cases and the cochleas only in both ears of 1 case.

The audiovestibuar manifestations, as reported in the literature, are somewhat different from those of polyarteritis nodosa in that the hearing losses are usually fluctuant and progressive over a period of months rather than sudden and profound, and vertigo is episodic and more severe. The inner ear pathology, on the other hand, is similar to that seen in polyarteritis nodosa but with more severe involvement of the vestibular system and more fibro-osseous proliferation.

It seems probable that the inner ear changes in Cogan's disease are caused by an immune response to proteins of the membranous labyrinth occurring in association with a nonorgan-specific autoimmune syndrome that also prominently involves the tissues of the eye and other organs. It is not clear what role, if any, obliterative vasculitis plays in the pathogenesis of the inner ear pathology in Cogan's syndrome.

Relapsing Polychondritis

Relapsing polychondritis is characterized by inflammatory reaction in multiple cartilages. Initial symptoms may consist of hyperemia and edematous auricles, joint pains, tender and swollen nasal septum, conjunctivitis, iritis, dyspnea, cough, fever, malaise, fatigue, hearing loss, and vertigo. Histological studies show that chondrocytes lose their cytoplasm until only nuclear remnants remain. Fibrous tissue replaces the destroyed and fragmented cartilage. At the interface of cartilage and fibrous tissue is an infiltrate of plasma cells and lymphocytes. There is a high incidence of associated autoimmune diseases as well as involvement of the vascular system, leading to valvular insufficiency, aneurysms, and focal or diffuse vasculitis.

Audiovestibular symptoms include hearing loss that can be bilateral or unilateral, conductive and/or sensorineural, sudden and profound in onset or rapidly (or slowly) progressive, and vertigo [10].

Hoshino et al. [11, 12] report a case of relapsing polychondritis with rapidly progressive bilateral hearing loss and vertigo 5 months after the onset of nasal symptoms (table 2). Examination revealed bilateral profound deafness and no response to ice water caloric tests in either ear. In spite of intensive steroid and immunosuppressive drug therapy the patient died 11 months after the onset of audiovestibular symptoms. The left ear was studied by scanning electron microscopy and the right ear by conventional serial sectioning for light microscopy (table 3). Histopathological findings in both ears included degeneration of the organs of Corti into mounds of flattened cells, deformation and partial encapsulation of the tectorial membranes, diffuse patchy atrophy of the striae vasculares, partial degeneration of the sensory epithelium of the maculas and cristas, and, in the right ear, fibrous proliferation and ossification in the scala tympani of the basal turn and lateral canal.

Because there is no cartilage in the inner ear, it can be assumed that the inner ear pathology is caused by obliterative vasculitis of the labyrinthine artery or its branches. The globuli interossei of the enchondral bony labyrinth consist of islands of calcified cartilage which probably would not generate an antigenic response. Furthermore, there is no evidence of pathologic changes in the enchondral bone of the right ear of the case presented by Hoshino et al. which had been prepared for light microscopic study.

Organ-Specific Autoimmune Inner Ear Disease

In 1979, McCabe [13] reported the first series of patients with progressive bilateral sensorineural hearing loss who were responsive to immunosuppressive therapy. Subsequently, he [14] and others [15, 16] have reported that autoimmune disease may cause a constellation of audiovestibular symptoms that may be sudden in onset or slowly progressive and that may have a unilateral or bilateral onset. The symptoms may mimic Ménière's disease with fluctuation of hearing and acute, severe vertiginous episodes with nausea and vomiting.

The diagnosis of autoimmune disease of the inner ear is based on a combination of clinical manifestations and laboratory tests; however, at this time there are no tests that provide unequivocal proof of the disease. Clinically, suspicion should be aroused with the presentation of hearing loss (unilateral or bilateral) and/or vertigo with loss of caloric response (unilateral or bilateral) that is progressive and without obvious cause, particularly, but not necessarily, when the symptoms are rapidly progressive. A general survey of humoral autoimmunity (antigen nonspecific tests) includes immunoglobulins (IgM, IgG, IgA), C-reactive protein (CRP) level in the serum, screening for rheumatoid factors and autoantibodies (antinuclear factor (ANA), antiperinuclear factor (APNF)), and a profile of the complement system.

In the complicated so-called antigen-specific tests, the blood of the patient is processed with inner ear tissues that are acquired from patients undergoing surgical removal of acoustic tumors or from autopsy specimens. The two tests that have been used, the leukocyte migration inhibition test [14] and the leukocyte transformation test [15], have shown good reliability in patients with strong clinical evidence of inner ear autoimmune disease. The most convincing support for the diagnosis of the disease is a positive therapeutic response to steroid and/or immunosuppressive therapy.

Case CK: In 1978 this 53-year-old male maintenance engineer felt dizzy and nauseated when arising in the morning. He was unable to stand. He vomited later in the morning as vertigo increased, and he became severely ataxic. He was hospitalized for diagnostic studies. Polytomography revealed normal temporal bones with normal-appearing internal auditory canals. Technetium brain scan and electrocardiogram were normal. Glucose was 100 mg, uric acid 5.9 mg, and cholesterol 162 mg. Hemoglobin was 16.1 g, hematocrit 46.4%, and the differential count was normal. Three-hour glucose tolerance test showed the following values: 87 mg at 1 h, 175 mg at 2 h, 166 mg at 3 h, and 161 mg at 4 h, and all urines were negative. It was noted at the time of this hospitalization that he was unsteady and that his gait was wide and unsure. He had difficulty standing on one leg and was very unsteady in the Romberg position. He had trouble touching his nose with his index finger. Upon discharge from the hospital he was given prescriptions for Dramamine and Antivert. The discharge diagnosis was Ménière's disease, diabetes mellitus, and cervical arthritis.

During 1978 and 1979, he continued to have episodic vertigo and noted a progressive loss of hearing in both ears. He stated that his hearing seemed to be worse after experiencing pain in the ears. The pain occurred primarily on the left, but also occasionally on the right. It was associated with a feeling of pressure in the ears, as well as increased sensitivity to sound.

In 1980, an ear, nose and throat examination revealed the tympanic membranes to appear normal, the tuning fork tests were normal, and the oral cavity revealed whitish submucosal patches. The mouth, pharynx, nasopharynx, larynx, and neck were otherwise negative. There was no spontaneous or positional nystagmus. Falling to the right was noted in the tandem Romberg position. An audiogram revealed a bilateral descending type sensorineural hearing loss that was worse in the left ear. There was moderate impairment of speech reception and discrimination scores in the left ear.

Electronystagmography showed right canal paresis. Tomograms of the temporal bones revealed normal internal auditory canals. A diagnosis of Ménière's disease was made again, and it was recommended that he avoid salt and caffeine, but that he continue the use of vitamins B and C and take Antivert 3 times/day.

During 1980–1983, he was examined by an otolaryngologist on numerous occasions. It was noted that he was allergic to Renograffin dye. He continued to have episodes of vertigo often associated with pain in his ears and complained of a pulsating tinnitus. Whitish plaques continued to appear on the mucous membranes of his oral cavity. On one occasion in 1980 he was noted to have a slow horizontal nystagmus to the left and tended to fall to the left. He was given a prescription for Lipoflavinoid to be taken 3 times/day. In 1981 he was noted to have a cholinergic urticaria which was treated with Atarax. In 1981 he was treated with steroids for his vertigo and hearing loss without improvement, and it was noted at that time that he had a persistent urticarial rash. He was also being medicated with digoxin for arrhythmia. During these years (1980–1983) repeat audiograms showed a steady progression of hearing loss in both ears (fig. 3). The speech reception thresholds progressed from 30 dB in 1980 to 60 dB in 1983, and speech discrimination dropped from 80–90% to 40–60%. In 1981 he began using a hearing aid in his right ear. An electronystagmogram in April 1981 revealed no spontaneous or positional nystagmus and no responses to the Fitzgerald-Hallpike caloric tests in either ear.

In 1981 an internist noted that his SMA-12 and SMAC-20 were normal. The blood count showed 12,500 white cells/ml^3 with 72 segs, 3 bands, and 25 lymphocytes. Hemoglobin was 16.1 g, hematocrit was 47.5%, and mean corpuscular volume was 90 μm^3. Platelet estimation was normal. Fasting blood sugar and 16:00 h sugars were all normal, although the patient's 5-hour glucose tolerance test had revealed values of 104 mg fasting, 210 mg at 1 h, 186 mg at 2 h, 96 mg at 3 h, 91 mg at 4 h, and 98 mg at 5 h. Erythrocyte sedimentation rate was slightly elevated at 16 mm (normal 1–13 mm/h). Prothrombin, partial prothrombin time, urinalysis, ANA titer, and immunoglobulins A, G, and M were normal. IgE fraction was elevated to 246 (normal below 175). Parathormone level was 1,200 (nor-

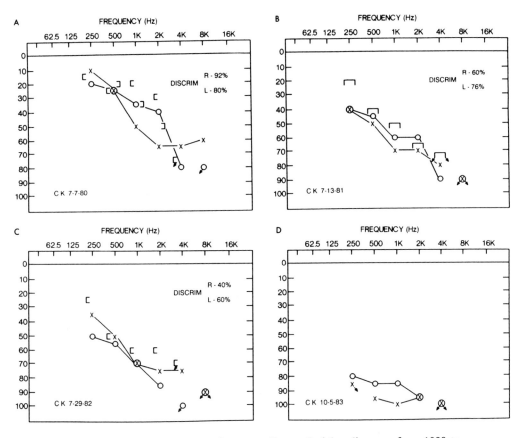

Fig. 3. Case CK, autoimmune inner ear disease. Serial audiograms from 1980 to 1983 showing progressive bilateral sensorineural hearing loss. For 2 years prior to his death in 1987 at age 63, he and his physicians considered him to be totally deaf.

mal 430–1,860). Leukocyte alkaline phosphatase was slightly elevated to 121. Doppler sonogram showed normal supraorbital flow. Electroencephalogram was within normal limits. Holter monitor showed up to 40 premature ventricular contractions per hour without coupling. Resting electrocardiogram showed occasional premature ventricular contractions in the vertical electrical position, and otherwise negative findings. Chest x-ray revealed prominence of the aortic knob and some minimal hypertrophic osteoarthritic change in the bony thorax. CT scan of the brain revealed normal findings. The patient was intermittently febrile during his hospital stay (tempadot method). His blood pressure averaged 115/80. The diagnoses made were: (1) Ménière's disease; (2) hypertensive cardiovascular disease; (3) premature ventricular contractions; (4) diabetes mellitus, and (5) bilateral Dupuytren's contracture of the hands.

In 1981 this man sought the opinion of another otolaryngologist concerning his progressive sensorineural hearing loss. This otolaryngologist diagnosed the condition as a progressive degenerative cochleovestibular process and recommended another course of steroid therapy. (It is quite clear that this consultant was thinking of autoimmune inner ear disease.)

In 1983 a neurological consultant summarized his findings as follows. 'The patient has a progressive hearing loss and repeated attacks of dizziness and drowsiness without nausea or vomiting that last for about 24 hours. Even between attacks he is never free of a sense of dizziness and it is increased in the dark. Intermittently there has been pain in the right mandible and right ear. He has an urticarial rash with itching that has been refractory to treatment. When walking, he experiences some "bouncing of lights". He describes a sensation of "locusts in his ears" during the attacks of vertigo. His medications include Lanoxin for irregular heart beat, meclizine for vertigo, and Tagamet for urticaria. The patient states that another CT scan of the head was reported to be negative. The cranial nerve functions are all within normal limits except for the VIIIth cranial nerve. There is no nystagmus in any position. There are no abnormal reflexes and strength is normal. The sensory functions are normal and his gait shows a wide base. There are areas of urticaria all over his body with raised levels of skin.' This neurologist agreed with the diagnosis of Ménière's disease but was unclear as to how to relate it to the urticaria.

In 1983, for compensation purposes, the patient was declared to be totally disabled because of bilateral profound sensorineural hearing loss and total loss of vestibular function.

The last entry in the medical records available to us was made again by the neurological consultant in 1986. 'The patient is now unable to work because of his hearing loss and poor equilibrium and because of insecurity in his gait. He is very unsteady in the dark, but denies any dizziness. He often awakens with headaches which improve after he has been up for a period of time. He weighs 135 pounds compared to 156 pounds three years previously. Again there are skin lesions which have seemingly baffled everybody so far. His blood pressure is 120/72. He has grade 3 pitting edema of lower legs. Except for the VIIIth nerve, all cranial nerves again show normal functions. There is no muscle weakness and no fasciculations or abnormalities of muscle tone. The muscle stretch reflexes are symmetrically present. As long as he can keep his eyes open, his gait is unremarkable but he is very unsteady on standing with his eyes closed. Sensory examination is normal. The weight loss is puzzling. The pancreas studies have been normal and there is no evidence to suggest a malabsorption syndrome.'

On November 7, 1987, at the age of 63, the patient died. Autopsy revealed bilateral bronchopneumonia, atherosclerosis of the coronary and renal arteries, septic splenitis, and fatty degeneration of the liver. The patient had pledged his temporal bones to the National Temporal Bone Bank and they were removed and placed in fixative solution 18 h after death.

Temporal bone pathology: The temporal bones are in an excellent state of preservation and preparation. During sectioning of the left temporal bone, a metallic prosthesis was encountered in the oval window. It was removed and identified as a Cody tack which had obviously been surgically introduced as a treatment for the vertiginous episodes. There is a slight inward surgical subluxation of the posterior margin of the footplate. The silhouette of the tack, now removed, extends through the footplate about 0.5 mm into the vestibule and is encapsulated by a multilayered fibrous sheath. The pathological findings are otherwise similar in the two ears and may be described together.

The mucosa of the middle ears and mastoids is slightly thickened by diffuse infiltration and focal aggregates of round cells. In some areas these aggregates of cells contain larger mononuclear cells probably representing macrophages. The smaller round cells appear to be a mixture of lymphocytes and plasma cells, the latter identified by their eccentrically located nuclei.

The bony labyrinths have a normal configuration; however, the enchondral layers show a large amount of bone without osteocytes. Remodelling into healthy-appearing lamellar bone is seen around vascular channels. Parts of the modiolus, particularly the areas around the spiral canal and the osseous spiral lamina, take a deep basophilic stain and also appear to be devoid of osteocytes (fig. 4).

The organs of Corti are in an advanced stage of degeneration (fig. 5). The outer hair cells are missing; however, some inner hair cells remain. Hensen's cells are present but flattened. The vessel of the tympanic lip and the vessel at the basilar membrane are enlarged and congested with blood. There are focal collections of lymphocytes and plasma cells within the tympanic lamellae and spiral ligaments. The tectorial membranes are

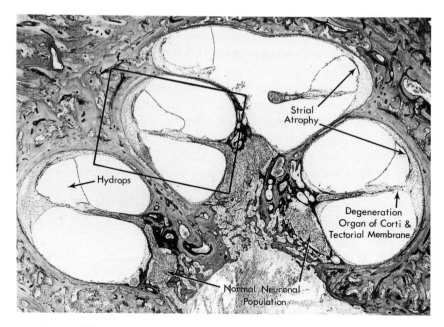

Fig. 4. Mid-modiolar section of the right cochlea showing diffuse degeneration of the organ of Corti, large patches of atrophy of the stria vascularis, extensive atrophy of the tectorial membrane including encapsulation in the apical region, endolymphatic hydrops, and focal distribution of basophilic staining of bone of the modiolus. The cochlear neuronal population appears normal. See figure 5.

shrunken throughout and partially encapsulated in the apical turns. The limbuses show loss of fibrocytes; however, the interdental cells are present. There is proliferation of fibrous tissue in the inner spiral tunnels. Reissner's membranes are moderately distended in all turns and appear to be thickened by an increased cellularity in both the mesothelial and epithelial cell layers. The striae vasculares show large areas of atrophy in all turns. There is a loose network of fibrous tissue seen in the inner part of the scalae vestibuli and scalae tympani of the first and second turns. There is a focal deposit of new bone in the scalae tympani of the basal turns located near the round windows (fig. 6). The cochlear neuronal populations including the dendrites appear to be normal.

The saccular walls are collapsed onto the maculas and are thickened by fibrous hyperplasia (fig. 7). Large areas of the sensory epithelia of the saccular maculas consist of an irregular layer of supporting cells with a few

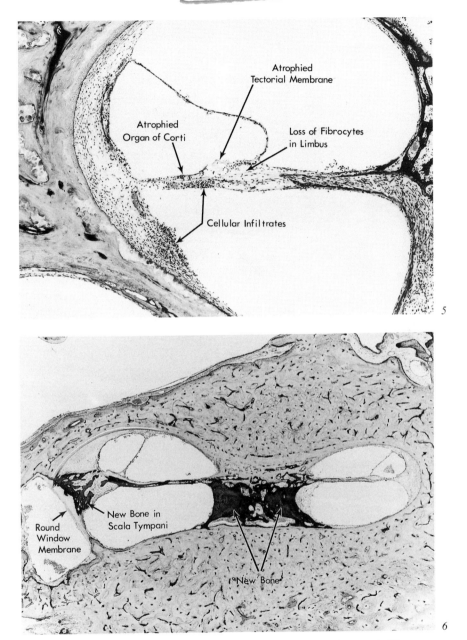

Fig. 5. Framed area in figure 4 showing focal cellular infiltrates in the spiral ligament and tympanic lamella, degeneration of the organ of Corti and tectorial membrane, endolymphatic hydrops, and loss of fibrocytes in the limbus.

Fig. 6. New bone and fibrous tissue in the scala tympani of the basal turn of the left cochlea.

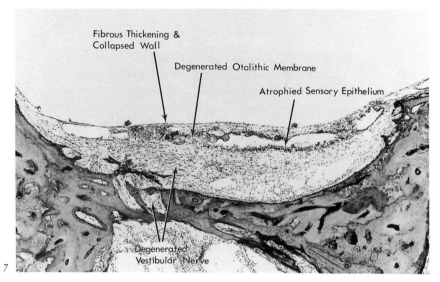

Fibrous Thickening &
Collapsed Wall

Degenerated Otolithic Membrane

Atrophied Sensory Epithelium

Degenerated
Vestibular Nerve

7

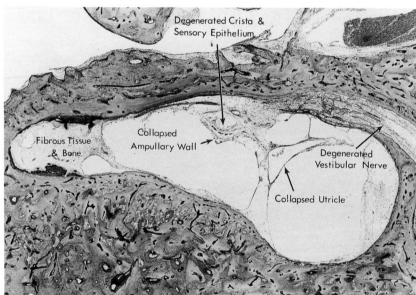

Degenerated Crista &
Sensory Epithelium

Fibrous Tissue
& Bone

Collapsed
Ampullary Wall

Degenerated
Vestibular Nerve

Collapsed Utricle

8

Fig. 7. Saccular macula of the right ear showing collapse and thickening of the saccular wall, degeneration of the otolithic membrane and sensory epithelium, and total loss
of vestibular nerve fibers.

Fig. 8. The ampullary wall and semicircular duct of the left lateral semicircular canal
are collapsed and degenerated. The crista, including the stroma and sensory epithelium, is
severely degenerated. Fibrous tissue and bone occupy the perilymphatic space of the
canal. The vestibular nerve is totally degenerated.

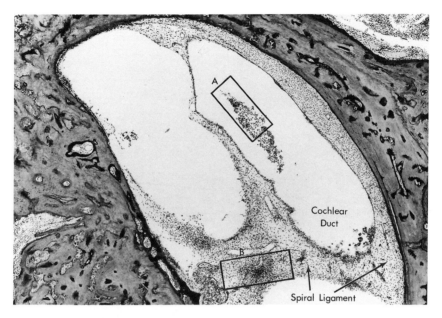

Fig. 9. Aggregates of perivascular cells in the spiral ligament and free-floating cells in the endolymph in the hook region of the basal turn of the right ear. See figure 10.

scattered hair cells. Bewteen the thick collapsed walls of the saccules and the degenerated sensory epithelia are collections of round and ovoid basophilic structures, some of which have coalesced into larger cystic spaces and which may represent the remains of degenerated otoconia as well as other amorphous debris. The utricular walls are partially collapsed and the sensory epithelia of the maculas contain some patches of supporting cells, but hair cells are missing. Most of the stroma of the utricular maculas is replaced by fibrous tissue which contains aggregates of lymphocytes and plasma cells as well as scattered basophilic inclusions.

All semicircular ducts and ampullas are collapsed and the cristas are severely degenerated with no sensory epithelium remaining (fig. 8). Loose fibrous tissue and some new bone occupy part of the semicircular canals and superior part of the vestibules.

There are focal infiltrates of lymphocytes and plasma cells in the posterior ampullary nerves, the gasserian ganglion, and in the cochlear and vestibular nerve trunks as well as in the endoneurium of the facial nerve.

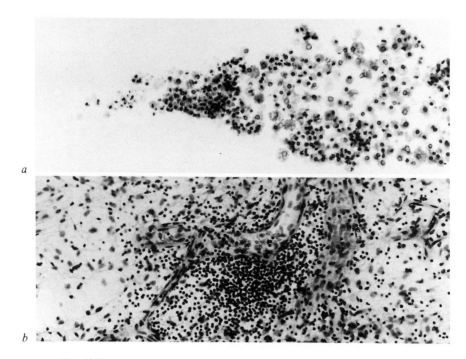

Fig. 10. Framed areas in figure 9. *a* These free-floating cells appear to be a mixture of lymphocytes, plasma cells, and macrophages. Some of the larger cells have a granular acidophilic cytoplasm resembling eosinophils. *b* This perivascular infiltrate consists predominantly of small round cells with sparse cytoplasm and centrally located nuclei and are presumed to be lymphocytes.

There are scattered focal aggregates of plasma cells, lymphocytes, and macrophages in the endolymphatic and perilymphatic spaces (fig. 9, 10). Bone fills the vestibular aqueduct of the right ear (fig. 11). The left internal carotid artery appears to be totally blocked by intimal proliferation.

Comment

The histological findings in the temporal bones of case CK are similar to those of previously reported cases of audiovestibular involvement occurring in association with systemic autoimmune diseases. The pathological features that characterize autoimmune inner ear disease are: (1) destruction of inner ear tissues including the sense organs, their supporting

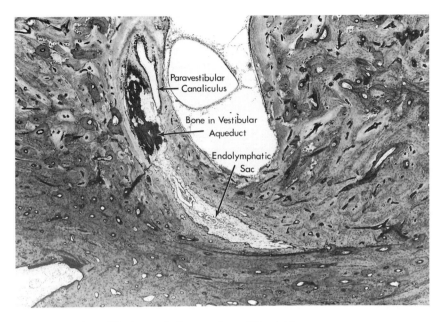

Fig. 11. Bone fills the vestibular aqueduct of the right ear.

structures, and eventually the membranous labyrinth; (2) scattered infiltrates and free-floating aggregates of lymphocytes, plasma cells, and macrophages, and (3) focal or diffuse proliferation of fibrous tissue and bone. Endolymphatic hydrops is a frequent but not constant finding.

In the case presented, the presence of an urticarial rash of several years' duration that was refractory to treatment may be viewed as further support for the diagnosis of an autoimmune disorder. The argument may be made that involvement of the skin and oral mucosa disqualifies this case as an organ-specific inner ear autoimmune disease. Furthermore, his recurring fever, progressive loss of weight, and eventual death can hardly be attributed to disease limited to the inner ears. Yet, his symptoms were so overwhelmingly of an audiovestibular nature that the inner ears were certainly the primary target organs for several years during the course of this man's presumed autoimmune disease.

The inner ear pathology is unique and when combined with the clinical manifestations cannot be mistaken for viral labyrinthitis (mumps, measles), sudden deafness, or Ménière's disease, the pathologies of which have been clearly described in previous reports.

References

1   Campbell SM, Montanaro A, Bardana EJ: Head and neck manifestations of autoimmune disease. Am J Otolaryngol 1983;4:187–216.

2   Gussen R: Polyarteritis nodosa and deafness. A human temporal bone study. Arch Otorhinolaryngol 1977;217:263–271.

3   Jenkins HA, Pollak AM, Fisch U: Polyarteritis nodosa as a cause of sudden deafness. A human temporal bone study. Am J Otolaryngol 1981;2:99–107.

4   Yanagita N, Yokoi H, Koide J, et al: Acute bilateral deafness with nephritis: a human temporal bone study. Laryngoscope 1987;97:345–352.

5   Yoon TH, Paparella MM, Schachern PA: Systemic vasculitis: a temporal bone histopathologic study. Laryngoscope 1989;99:600–609.

6   Schuknecht HF: Pathology of the Ear. Cambridge, Harvard University Press, 1974.

7   Fisher ER, Hellstrom HF: Cogan's syndrome and systemic vascular disease. Analysis of pathologic features with reference to its relationship to thromboangiitis obliterans (Buerger). Arch Pathol 1961;72:572–592.

8   Wolff D, Bernhard WG, Tsutsumi S, et al: The pathology of Cogan's syndrome causing profound deafness. Ann Otol Rhinol Laryngol 1965;74:507–520.

9   Rarey KE, Bicknell JM, Davis LE: Intralabyrinthine osteogenesis in Cogan's syndrome. Am J Otolaryngol 1986;4:387–390.

10   Cody DTR, Sones DA: Relapsing polychondritis: audiovestibular manifestations. Laryngoscope 1971;81:1208–1222.

11   Hoshino T, Kato I, Kodama A, et al: Sudden deafness in relapsing polychondritis. Acta Otolaryngol (Stockh) 1978;86:418–427.

12   Hoshino T, Ishii T, Kodama A, et al: Temporal bone findings in a case of sudden deafness and relapsing polychondritis. Acta Otolaryngol (Stockh) 1980;90:257–261.

13   McCabe BF: Autoimmune sensorineural hearing loss. Ann Otol Rhinol Laryngol 1979;88:585–589.

14   McCabe BF: Autoimmune inner ear disease: clinical varieties of presentation: in Veldman JE, McCabe BF (eds): Otoimmunology. Amsterdam, Kugler Publications, 1987, chapt 15, pp 143–148.

15   Hughes GB, Kinney SE, Barna BP, et al: Autoimmune inner ear disease. Laboratory tests and audio-vestibular treatment responses; in Veldman JE, McCabe BF (eds): Otoimmunology. Amsterdam, Kugler Publications, 1987, chapt 16, pp 149–155.

16   Veldman JE: Immune-mediated inner ear disorders. New syndromes and their etiopathogenesis; in Veldman JE, McCabe BF (eds): Otoimmunology. Amsterdam, Kugler Publications, 1987, chapt 14, pp 125–141.

Harold F. Schuknecht, MD, Department of Otolaryngology, Massachusetts Eye and Ear Infirmary, 243 Charles Street, Boston, MA 02114 (USA)

Pfaltz CR, Arnold W, Kleinsasser O (eds): Bearing of Basic Research on Clinical
Otolaryngology. Adv Otorhinolaryngol. Basel, Karger, 1991, vol 46, pp 71–77

Immune-Mediated Inner Ear Disorders:
An Otoimmunologist's View

Jan E. Veldman

Department of Otorhinolaryngology, University of Utrecht, The Netherlands

Otologists start to recognize that immunological mechanisms can play
an important role in the pathogenesis of different inner ear disorders.
Otoimmunology – immunology of the ear and related structures – progress
[1–3]. Sensorineural hearing disorders, which are today still categorized as
rapidly progressive sensorineural hearing loss of unknown etiology, sudden
deafness and Ménière's disease comprise patients in whom immune mechanisms play occasionally a central role in the development of the disease.

Our knowledge of the pathways of an immune response in and around
the inner ear is still limited but gradually developing [1–4]. Much of what
is known today about inner ear immunity comes from animal models; the
human inner ear remains inaccessible for immunological studies in clinical
otology. Temporal bone studies from patients with immune-mediated sensorineural hearing loss disorders are rare and mainly limited to a few cases
of Cogan's syndrome. Newly developed immunohistology has never been
applied yet to such temporal bone studies.

Schuknecht [5] introduces his well-known book 'Pathology of the Ear'
as follows: 'A thorough knowledge of pathophysiology forms the basis for
intelligent and successful prevention and management of successful prevention and management of disease. The source of such knowledge derives
principally from laboratory research performed by individuals who are
trained in scientific methodology. By compiling the most significant facts
from basic and clinical science and bringing them together with clinical
expertise, one may create ideal circumstances for further progress.'

I do hope that this contribution meets the above criteria. Its contents,
however, are restricted to the presently best defined immune-mediated

sensorineural hearing loss syndromes which are associated with systemic autoimmune diseases [1, 7, 8]. In addition, the process of applying newly developed immunotechnology to the microdissected human temporal bone is illustrated by means of intermediate-sized filament protein analyses of the inner ear cytoskeleton [12]. Through this method optimal postmortem preservation of antigenic sites in the human inner ear is documented. It hopefully adds to a new venue for immunohistopathology of the ear, also of those rare cases with immune-mediated audio-vestibular dysfunction.

Autoimmunity and the Inner Ear

The etiology of autoimmunity is not clear. Autoreactivity may be the consequence of a breakdown of an individual's immunological homeostasis, in which regulatory mechanisms prevent the stimulation of self-reactive lymphocytes. An autoimmune immunologic response may follow a preceding tissue injury: antigens that were sequestered within the organ and lacked previous contact with the immune apparatus are thus released and immune reactivity may occur (e.g. certain eye diseases). Antigens may also be modified by drugs or viruses resulting in a new antigen of nonself character giving rise to autoimmune reactivity. Furthermore, certain microorganisms carry antigenic determinants which are identical to the antigenic make-up of human tissues; immune responses occur against the invader and subsequently cross-reactivity gives rise to a tissue injury (streptococci → heart and kidney). Genetic factors seem to play a role in the development of autoimmune diseases. HLA association with disorders of autoimmune character has been established over the past years.

Autoimmunity presents itself clinically in a certain line. At one end, organspecific diseases with circulating organspecific autoantibodies or T cells (e.g. Hashimoto's thyroiditis), in the center of this line, organ diseases limited to one organ but with nonorgan-specific circulating auto-antibodies (e.g. primary biliary cirrhosis) and at the other end, systemic nonorgan-specific diseases with circulating auto-antibodies of various specificities (e.g. rheumatoid arthritis, SLE, Sjögren's syndrome). Immune-mediated audiovestibular dysfunctioning is somewhere located along this line. It may stand by itself [6] or the inner ear can be one of the targets in a more generalized systemic autoimmune disease [7, 8].

Clinical Otology

What is the clinical evidence for immunologic reactivity in audiovestibular disorders? This prompts three questions: (1) Does cochlear autoimmune sensorineural hearing loss with or without vertigo exist as a disease entity per se without further clinical and pathological expression of the disease at other sites? (2) How strong are the arguments that in cases with generalized autoimmune diseases also the inner ear is involved as one of the target organs and if so is the clinical behavior and treatment response identical as in the cases where only the inner ear is involved? (3) Is retrocochlear immunopathology present as an autoimmune phenomenon also being responsible for audiovestibular dysfunctioning?

In this collection of essays, Harris and Hughes have extensively dealt with the first issue. This contribution is focused on the two other questions.

In generalized autoimmune diseases vasculitis frequently occurs. It is considered to be caused by the deposition of circulating (auto-)immune complexes in vessel walls, followed by complement activation and the invasion of polymorphonuclear and monunuclear leukocytes. Vasculitis with immune complex deposition may result in complement depletion in the circulation. It should be noted that demonstration of circulating immune complexes is not equal to the diagnosis autoimmune vasculitis. Immune complexes can also be demonstrated in the circulation during infectious diseases or malignancies. A general survey for the presence of humoral autoimmunity includes the assessment of the sedimentation rate, serum immunoglobulins and CRP level, screening for rheumatoid factors, autoantibodies (ANF, SMA, APNF), circulating immune complexes and a full complement profile. If tissue biopsies of certain organ systems are difficult or impossible to obtain (inner ear), as in cases of suspected immune-mediated sensorineural hearing loss, biopsies of other organs may reveal the sequelae of a systemic autoimmune reaction (vasculitis). Radioisotope scintigraphy with gallium citrate (^{67}Ga) – which binds to leukocytes and detects in this way an inflammatory process – may help as a guiding tool for the site of a biopsy [7].

An immune complex-mediated autoimmune vasculitis leads to a flat bilateral threshold drop over all frequencies [7]. Generally both ears are involved. In our experience vestibular symptoms are rare. There is not always tinnitus. The hearing loss may develop both rapidly (in days or weeks) but also slowly (in months) progressive. Normal hearing returns often after short (1–2 weeks) corticosteroid treatment and remains stable afterwards without further medication. In our experience such cases do not need immunosuppressive cyclophosphamide treatment.

Circulating autoantibodies against neural tissue can play an important role in a rapidly progressive neuropathy, which may include audiovestibular dysfunctioning. A well-documented case was earlier published [8]: both vestibular and brain stem auditory evoked response testing indicated retrocochlear pathology, although all routine clinical immunology tests were negative. However, the patient's serum samples were positive for cross-reacting autoantibodies when tested on human temporal bone sections of an unrelated individual according to Arnold's method [9]. Spiral ganglion cells stained heavily positive. Rapid medical (corticosteroid) treatment brought this bilateral sensorineural deafness and vestibular dysfunction without tinnitus back to nearly normal levels within 2 weeks.

Immunohistology and the Adult Human Inner Ear

Immunohistology is an outstanding tool for function-structure relations in immune-mediated temporal bone disorders. The technique complements the morphology and allows a further distinction of cells, cell reactivity and cell identity at a microscopical level. Cells which are morphologically identical possess for instance cell membrane markers and cytoskeletal constituents which are unique for their specific function. Antibodies with a monospecificity are now used to distinguish and visualize such sites from each other. Even tissue origin and specificity can be determined [1–3]. Immunohistochemical studies of the human inner ear have remained scarce due to problems in applying routine immmunohistological techniques to the temporal bone. It is one factor that determines a lack of information on immune-mediated inner ear disorders today. Ear pathology research in this respect has still to be learned and taught [10–12].

Cryostat sectioning would be ideal to preserve optimal antigenicity but is for the human temporal bone not well applicable. Chemical fixation cannot be avoided, unfortunately. Since the human inner ear is surrounded by the bony labyrinth, prolonged decalcification prior to sectioning has always been considered to be inevitable. Both such processing steps can alter the antigenicity of any tissue considerably and may easily lead to false-negative results. Therfore, as a first step to develop a reliable processing technique for the human inner ear, a new procedure has been developed. It essentially consists of intralabyrinthine perfusion fixation immediately after death with microsurgical removal of the bony labyrinth prior to cryostat sectioning, so as to avoid the immunocompromising step of prolonged chemical decalcification. Recent investigations have shown that there are different fixatives which appear to be suitable for immunohistology of the inner ear [13]. It is, however, important to note that the choice of fixative depends on what kind of antigenic site is to be detected. Furthermore, the duration of fixation is important. Antigens will leach when fixation is too short. Overfixation may cause denaturation of antigens. As an example of this immunotechnique intermediate filament protein staining was performed. Antigenic sites of cytoskeletal proteins are highly susceptible for tissue fixation and therefore a subtle mirror for how adequate a processing technique has been performed for maintenance of original antigenicity. This holds in particular when monoclonal antibodies are used. Immunostaining with monoclonal antibodies to cytokeratins occurred in all epithelial cells along the cochlear duct and vestibular labyrinth, including most supporting cells of the organ of Corti, macula sacculi, macula utriculi and crista ampullaris. The details of this technical approach with its results were recently published by Bauwens et al. [12, 15, 16].

Problem-Solving in Autoimmune Inner Ear Disease

In this respect three issues are important to analyze: (1) A reliable animal model is needed to examine the concept whether the inner ear can be a target under experimental autoimmune conditions. Audiovestibular dysfunctioning should be demonstrated in relation to autoimmune inner ear injuries in a time sequence study. To prove the concept of autoimmunity it would be ideal if the disease appears to be transferable with hyperimmune serum, soluble products from the circulation or circulating lymphoid cells from one animal to another. Solid evidence is accumulating that the inner ear can be involved in an organ-specific autoimmune injury [see Harris, this volume]. The involvement of the inner ear in systemic autoimmune diseases still comes from clinical observations only, but is quite feasible since experimental analyses have proven that the cochlea is not an immunoprivileged site for either active or passive transfer of immunoglobulins and/or lymphoid cells from the circulation into the inner ear compartment [1–3]. (2) The characterization of a specific autoantibody (antibodies) or T cells directed against inner ear structures needs further laboratory research. Recent data indicate that both patients and animals with progressive autoimmune sensorineural hearing loss have a specific anticochlear antibody in their circulation [14]. However, it still has to be determined whether the antigenic epitope against which the antibody is directed is unique for the inner ear or even the cochlea. Up to now, cell-mediated immunity has never been demonstrated to be operational in this autoimmune condition. (3) Immunohistological evaluation should be added to routine temporal bone studies from patients suspected of immune-mediated inner ear disease whenever such specimens become available. Postmortem tissue handling needs to be adapted to serve this purpose. Immediate postmortem tissue handling through intralabyrinthine perfusion fixation with carefully determined solutions, specimen dissection for cryostat techniques, microslicing of the temporal bone and even plastic embedding with nonimmune compromising monomers are all steps forward in a process of applying newly developed immuno- and biotechnology to temporal bone research [10–16].

References

1 Veldman JE, McCabe BF (eds): Otoimmunology. Amsterdam/Berkeley, Kugler Publications, 1987.

2 Veldman JE, et al (eds): Immunobiology, Autoimmunity, Transplantation in Otorhinolaryngology. Amsterdam/Berkeley, Kugler Publications, 1985.

3 Veldman JE (ed): Immunobiology, Histophysiology, tumorimmunology in Otorhinolaryngology. Amsterdam/Berkeley, Kugler Publications, 1987.

4 Harris JP: Experimental immunology of the inner ear; in Pfaltz CR, Arnold W, Kleinsasser O (eds): Bearing of Basic Research on Clinical Otolaryngology. Adv Otorhinolaryngol. Basel, Karger, 1991, vol 46, pp 26–33.

5 Schuknecht HF: Pathology of the Ear. Cambridge, Harvard University Press, 1974.

6 McCabe BF: Autoimmune sensorineural hearing loss. Ann Otol Rhinol Laryngol 1979;88:585.

7 Veldman JE, Roord JJ, O'Connor AF, Shea JJ: Autoimmunity and inner ear disorders. An immune complex mediated sensorineural hearing loss. Laryngoscope 1984; 94:501.

8 Veldman JE: Cochlear and retrocochlear immune-mediated inner ear disorders. Pathogenetic mechanisms and diagnostic tools. Ann Otol Rhinol Laryngol 1986;95: 535.

9 Arnold W, Pfaltz CR, Altermatt HJ: Evidence of serum antibodies against inner ear tissues in the blood of patients with certain sensorineural disorders. Acta Otolaryngol (Stockh) 1987;103:373.

10 Veldman JE, Meeuwsen F, Van Dijk M, Key Q, Huizing EH: Progress in temporal bone histopathology II. Immunotechnology applied to the temporal bone. Acta Otolaryngol (Stockh) 1985 (suppl 423):29.

11 Veldman JE, Meeuwsen F, Huizing EH: Advances in otoimmunology: New trends in functional pathology of the temporal bone. Laryngoscope 1987;97:413.

12 Bauwens LJJM, Veldman JE, Huizing EH: Progress in temporal bone histopathology. III. An improved technique for immunohistochemical investigation of the adult human inner ear. Acta Otolaryngol (Stockh) 1990 (suppl 470):34.

13 Altermatt HJ, Gebbers JO, Arnold W, Kraft R, Laissue JA: Preparation of human temporal bone for immunohistochemical investigation. ORL 1989;51:83.

14 Harris JP, Sharp PA: Inner ear autoantibodies in patients with rapidly progressive sensorineural hearing loss. Laryngoscope 1990;100:516.

15 Bauwens LJJM: Intermediate filaments in the adult human audio-vestibular organ. PhD Thesis. University of Utrecht, 1991.

16 Bauwens LJJM, Veldman JE: Intermediate filaments in the adult human inner ear; in McCabe BF, Veldman JE, Harris JP, Lim DJ, Mogi G (eds): Immunobiology in Otology, Rhinology and Laryngology. Amsterdam/Berkeley, Kugler-Ghedini Publications, 1991.

Jan E. Veldman, MD, PhD, Department of Otorhinolaryngology,
University Hospital Utrecht, Heidelberglaan 100,
NL–3584 CX Utrecht (The Netherlands)

Pfaltz CR, Arnold W, Kleinsasser O (eds): Bearing of Basic Research on Clinical
Otolaryngology. Adv Otorhinolaryngol. Basel, Karger, 1991, vol 46, pp 78–81

Autoimmune Inner Ear Disease:
Results of Therapy

Brian F. McCabe

Department of Otolaryngology, The University of Iowa, Iowa City, Iowa, USA

We have accumulated a series of 72 patients to the present time with a
relatively uncommon form of progressive bilateral sensorineural deafness
which responds to immunosuppression. Although relatively uncommon, it
is important to recognize for it is one of the few forms of sensorineural
deafness for which we have a treatment. Our initial term suggested for this
condition was *autoimmune sensorineural hearing loss* [1]. We now know
that not only the cochlear compartment but the vestibular compartment
may be involved as well, hence, *autoimmune inner ear disease* (AIED) is
the more appropriate designation for the condition [2].

When the vestibular compartment is involved as well, the symptom
set will usually manifest itself as quite different from Ménière's disease.
These patients have vertigo in spells similar to Ménière's disease, but they
have them in storms – many in a day rather than one or two per week or
per month. Also, they are not asymptomatic between spells but subjective-
ly, or objectively, ataxic between spells. Patients with Ménière's disease are
asymptomatic between spells except for the deafness. These differences
will help the otologist distinguish between the two [3].

In terms of treatment of AIED, the cornerstone is cyclophosphamide,
and not prednisone [4]. I urge that the latter not be used as sole treatment,
or even a test of treatment, because too many patients who actually have
the disease will be missed, and their hearing will irretrievably be lost.
Patients who progress to total deafness gain no benefit from treatment
once reaching that point. Patients on the other hand who have severe loss

improve to moderate loss, or from moderate loss to mild loss, or from mild loss to normal hearing. The most important gain in patients with severe loss is improvement in discrimination scores enabling them to be rehabilitated with hearing aids (e.g., improvements of 40–50%). These are the goals of treatment and can in most cases be attained. In some patients we have been satisfied to arrest the progression of the hearing loss, that is, put a 'floor' under the deafness, long-term.

Most patients in our series are in the 30- to 50-year age bracket. The youngest is 16 years and the oldest 64 years. This generally fits within the age envelope of other autoimmune diseases.

Since we do not have any unequivocal laboratory test for this disease, our practice is a test of treatment. This is not as specific a test as, let us say, a tissue biopsy, but it is as good a test as a glucose tolerance test for diabetes mellitus in that it is specific for that particular patient.

The test of treatment is the administration of cyclophosphamide 60 mg (or 2 mg/kg) every 12 h and prednisone 30 mg every other day, for 4 weeks. These doses are relatively small in terms of side effects but adequate for treatment. If then any significant increase in pure tones or discrimination on audiometry (average 15 dB in any three frequencies or more than 20% discrimination score) the test of treatment is positive and full treatment is commenced.

Full treatment consists of continuance of the same drugs and levels for 3 months. Then the cyclophosphamide is stopped and the prednisone continued for 2 weeks. If the hearing holds, the prednisone is tapered over 2 weeks. If hearing drops before or after the taper, full treatment is reinstituted for an additional 3 months. The same is then repeated if necessary.

We have had to treat some patients for as many as eight such cycles (2 years) but no longer than that. At such time, the autoimmune process appears to be burned out, or the pathophysiologic mechanism that brought about the attack upon the labyrinth has been reversed. In 3 patients who developed steroid toxicity and also uncontrollable white count drops, plasmapheresis was instituted with benefits [5].

It should be noted that 25% of our patients subsequently came down with other autoimmune diseases. This points to a fundamental immune diathesis in a significant number of these patients, far in excess of that seen in the public at large.

The most important message I wish to present is that cyclophosphamide, not prednisone, is the cornerstone of treatment of this disease. AIED is exquisitely sensitive to that drug, just as Wegner's granulomatosis, another autoimmune disease.

And yet, otologists are in the main reluctant to use the drug because it is not one they use frequently and apparently are not comfortable with it. Each however has a doctoral degree in medicine, can read and apply the Physician's Desk Reference, and has no difficulty using new drugs as they emerge. As stated above, a significant number of patients with this disease will be missed with prednisone treatment alone, to eventually lose all their hearing. Cyclophosphamide in a dosage of 2 mg/kg is quite safe if the usual precaution is observed, i.e., monitoring the white blood cell count. It should be taken weekly, and if it drops to 4,000/mm^3 the drug is stopped until it goes above 5,000, usually a few weeks. Actually this seldom happens because of the concomitant prednisone, which promotes a leukocytosis of polymorphonucleocytes but not killer lymphocytes. This is its chief role in the treatment program for AIED, not its immunosuppressant activity in which it is relatively weak. The complications of cyclophosphamide have been few and not threatening to life. The most common is scalp hair loss in women, occurring in 12% of patients to a significant degree (e.g., requiring use of a wig). In each case the hair has regrown after cessation of therapy. Only 1 patient had a significant infection, a carbuncle of the upper leg which required two surgical procedures to eliminate it. It is difficult to incriminate Cytoxan in this because all through the infection the white blood cell count was between 4,000 and 6,000/mm^3.

Conclusions

Autoimmune inner ear disease is a relatively uncommon disorder of the labyrinth, but an important one because it is one of the few such diseases for which we have a treatment. The best results are with a combination of moderate dosage cyclophosphamide and low dose prednisone. Results are gratifying, with significant improvement of hearing in the majority and cessation of progress of hearing in the rest who have the disease. We cannot unequivocally diagnose the disease pretreatment. Treatment over a period of 3–24 months has been necessary. Complications have been minor and few. It is a disease of young and early middle-aged adults for the most part. The clinician should be aware of the emergence of other autoimmune diseases, which will occur in probably one of four.

References

1   McCabe BF: Autoimmune sensorineural hearing loss. Ann Otol Rhinol Laryngol 1979;88:585–589.
2   McCabe BF: Autoimmune inner ear disease; in Bernstein J, Ogra P (eds): Immunology of the Ear. New York, Raven Press, 1987, pp 427–435.
3   McCabe BF: Autoimmune inner ear disease: Clinical varieties of presentation; in Veldman JE, McCabe BF (eds): Oto-Immunology. Amsterdam, Kugler Publications, 1987, pp 143–148.
4   McCabe BF: Autoimmune inner ear disease: therapy. Am J Otol 1989;10:196–197.
5   Luetje CM: Theoretical and practical implications for plasmapheresis in autoimmune inner ear disease. Laryngoscope 1989;99:1137–1146.

Brian F. McCabe, MD, Department of Otolaryngology – Head and Neck Surgery, The University of Iowa, Iowa City, IA 52242 (USA)

Pfaltz CR, Arnold W, Kleinsasser O (eds): Bearing of Basic Research on Clinical
Otolaryngology. Adv Otorhinolaryngol. Basel, Karger, 1991, vol 46, pp 82–91

Autoimmune Inner Ear Disease: Fact or Fantasy?

Gordon B. Hughes[a], Barbara P. Barna[b]

[a] Department of Otolaryngology and Communicative Disorders and
[b] Department of Immunopathology, The Cleveland Clinic Foundation,
Cleveland, Ohio, USA

For more than 30 years, researchers in Japan and (West) Germany
have studied autoimmune (immune-mediated) inner ear disease. Autoimmunity implies that inner ear proteins are recognized immunologically as
foreign or nonself. Lehnhardt [1] in 1958 reported cases of bilateral sensorineural hearing loss which he believed to result from anticochlear antibodies. Kikuchi [2] in 1959 described 'sympathetic otitis' with hearing loss
in the opposite ear following surgery on the other ear. Beichert [3] studied
histological autoimmune reactions in the cochlea in 1961. Terayama and
Yukihiro [4] in 1963 reported hearing loss in guinea pigs following immunization with homologous cochlea in Freund's adjuvant.

Because the putative inner ear antigens are not yet known, some clinicians still doubt that autoimmune inner ear disease exists. For this reason, presently we prefer the term 'immune-mediated' disease, and believe
the diagnosis is based on relatively distinct clinical manifestations, positive immune laboratory tests, and beneficial treatment response, as proposed by McCabe [5] in 1979. At the Cleveland Clinic Foundation over the
past 10 years, 101 patients have been diagnosed, 47 of whom have sufficient follow-up to judge treatment results [6]. These 47 patients can be
divided into two general diagnostic groups: those with suspicious clinical
manifestations and with positive lymphocyte transformation test (LTT)
results, and those with Cogan's syndrome. Cogan's syndrome consists of
ocular inflammation, immune inner ear disease, and negative blood test
for syphilis. Because the vestibuloauditory dysfunction of Cogan's syn-

drome, by definition, is immune-mediated, the LTT is less important. However, since Cogan's syndrome is rare and most patients with immune inner ear disease have no visible external findings, the LTT has been most important in diagnosing the majority of patients. In this report, we present our current experience with immune inner ear disease, with particular attention to laboratory diagnosis.

Laboratory Diagnosis

Immune laboratory tests are used to confirm a presumptive clinical diagnosis. Although the natural history of immune inner ear disease is not known, we believe that disease activity waxes and wanes. Furthermore, steroids and cytotoxic drugs suppress immune reactivity. Therefore, patients should be tested when symptoms are acute and immunotherapy is not being given. In general, tests are antigen-specific or antigen-nonspecific. Antigen-specific tests employ homologous or heterologous inner ear tissues which presumably contain the putative antigen(s), and search for cellular or humoral (antibody) activity as direct evidence of immune activity. Antigen-nonspecific tests do not employ inner ear tissues, and search for soluble circulating immune complexes as indirect evidence of immune activity.

Antigen-specific cellular immune tests include the LTT (blast) and migration inhibition test (MIT). Both tests assume that circulating lymphocytes which have immunlogic memory (i.e. specifically sensitized lymphocytes) identify the putative inner ear antigen(s) and thus undergo anamnestic responses in vitro. When a previously sensitized lymphocyte receives a second similar antigen exposure, a series of lymphocyte peptides, called lymphokines, is elaborated. The consequences of lymphokine activity can be detected by measuring blast transformation or migration inhibition.

Inner ear membranes first are obtained from patients during translabyrinthine surgery, unrelated to immune disease, without jeopardizing the welfare of any patient. These membranes are intact and presumably contain the antigens which incite immune inner ear disease.

A sterile tissue homogenate of these pooled membranes from 3–6 individuals is made in the laboratory, using at least four different dilutions of inner ear membrane extracts at protein concentrations ranging from 1.0 to 1,000 µg/ml. As a positive control for each test, leukocytes are challenged with a nonspecific mitogen, phytohemagglutinin, to confirm cellular competence of the leukocytes. Baseline reactivity in each test is obtained by incubating mononuclear cells with tissue media devoid of any antigen or mitogen. Nonspecific toxicity or antigenicity of extracts is screened by initial testing against leukocytes of 3 normal donors. Extracts showing such reactivity are discarded. Thereafter, specimens from various normal individuals are tested monthly as part of an established quality control program. Patient leukocytes in excess of those needed for immediate testing have proven to retain positivity after retrieval from cryogenic storage. Such specimens are helpful in checking activity of new batches of extracts. In addition, overall activity of patient leukocytes with extracts is plotted yearly. A survey of testing against six different extracts over a period of several years has indicated that extracts are not usable longer than 6 months. The overall mean incidence of positive tests was 17% (104/613 tests) with a range of 13–25% per month during a 6-month period. Thereafter, incidence of positive tests dropped sharply to 3% at 7 months or longer storage.

From a patient with suspicious signs and symptoms, a sample of whole, fresh blood is obtained when symptoms are active and the patient is not taking immunosuppressant medication. Mononuclear leukocytes are separated from the patient's blood by Ficoll-Hypaque centrifugation.

In the LTT [7], cells are mixed with inner ear proteins in microtiter plates for 7 days, with exposure to tritiated thymidine during the last 20 h. Each variable is tested in four replicate wells. Cells are harvested on filter paper and content of radiolabel determined in a liquid scintillation counter. Responses (incorporation of labelled thymidine) are determined by Student's t test comparing mean counts per minute (cpm) in cells exposed to medium alone with cells exposed to antigen. Interpretation of patient responses as normal or elevated ('positive') is done when $p < 0.05$ and when the stimulation index (antigen cpm/control cpm) exceeds normal range (0.7–1.5) rather than an arbitrary cutoff point. Normal control data are statistically determined from assays carried out on 50 normal hospital employees. The normal range represents two standard deviations above and below the normal mean (1.14).

This analysis produces three test interpretations: positive, borderline and negative. Because testing is performed in suspect (as opposed to random) patients, all positive results are interpreted as true positives. The records of all borderline patients are reviewed carefully. If clinical manifestations are suspicious or a treatment trial is beneficial, such results also are considered positive. Patients with Cogan's syndrome, by definition, have immune inner ear disease and are not always tested. The Cleveland Clinic Foundation laboratory was the first to utilize the LTT in immune inner ear disease [8]. At present it is our only diagnostic test.

McCabe [5] was the first to use the MIT in immune inner ear disease but now prefers a test battery because the MIT alone may not b sufficiently specific. In the MIT [9], capillary tubes are filled with mononuclear leukocytes and placed in chambers containing the various reagents outlined above. Three replicate chambers are used for each variable. After 24 h, areas of cell migration out of the capillary tubes are measured and mean and standard deviations are determined. A response is considered positive if migration areas in the presence of antigen are significantly different (p < 0.05 by t test) from those of controls containing medium alone.

Antigen-specific humoral immune tests include indirect immunofluorescence, enzyme-linked immunoassay (ELISA), and Western blot analysis. Indirect immunofluorescence techniques vary. Thin section temporal bone slices from humans or animals are used because membranes from translabyrinthine surgery are dessicated during removal. Frozen sections are incubated with appropriate dilutions of patient serum, followed by fluorescein-conjugated antibody to human immunoglobulin. Samples are then evaluated microscopically using a fluorescent microscope. Negative controls consist of labelled reagent alone, as well as sera from healthy individuals. Sera containing antinuclear antibodies from patients with lupus erythematosus are used as positive controls. Using immunofluorescence in temporal bone substrates, Arnold and co-workers [10, 11] found inner ear specific autoantibodies in 54 % of patients. Soliman [12] found specific autoantibodies in 18 % of patients. Veldman [13] identified reaction against the spiral ganglia. Elies and Plester [14] identified nonspecific reaction against nuclei, mitochondria, smooth muscle, vascular endothelium, sarcolemma and laminin in patients with various cochleovestibular disorders, compared with controls.

ELISA is performed using microtiter plates coated with 5 µg extract protein. Similar procedures have been reported previously in detail [15]. Coated plates are incubated with patient or control sera and then with alkaline phosphatase-labelled anti-human IgG (many other enzyme systems are used in clinical laboratory testing). Enzyme substrate (*p*-nitrophenyl phosphate) is added after plates have been washed free of unbound antibody. The enzyme reaction is stopped after 30 min with 3 *N* NaOH, and the color change measured spectrophotometrically at 405 nm in an

ELISA plate reader. Data are expressed as absorbance units, and patient and control sera are compared by t test with difference probability of less than 0.05 considered significant. Orozco et al. [16] used ELISA to study disease in guinea pigs and mice after cross-immunization with chick cochlear tissue. Their results will be published shortly.

In the Western blot technique of Harris and Sharp [17], 750 µg of inner ear extract from fresh bovine temporal bones are electrophoresed on a 5–17% SDS polyacrylamide gel for 4 h. Proteins are transferred to nitrocellulose using a Hoeffer transfer electrophoresis chamber for 2 h, and the nitrocellulose is then cut into strips. Human sera are diluted 1:1,000 and incubated overnight with the nitrocellulose strips. The strips are then rinsed and incubated for 1 h at 25 °C with a secondary rabbit anti-guinea pig immunoglobulin G (IgG) or rabbit anti-human IgG. They are then rinsed and incubated 1 h at 25 °C with ^{125}I staphylococcal protein A. The rinsed strips are dried, laid on Whatman blotter paper, and placed on Kodak X-Omat RP X-ray film with an intensifier screen. The film is developed after an overnight exposure at –70 °C.

Harris and Sharp [17] used Western blot analysis to study 54 patients with progressive sensorineural hearing loss and 14 normal controls. Nineteen (35%) of the hearing loss group showed a single or double band migrating at 68,000 molecular weight, differing significantly (p = 0.031) from one normal control (7%) who showed a similar band.

Antigen-nonspecific tests include cryoprecipitation (quantitative and qualitative), complement system (C1q binding, CH_{50}), autoantibodies (antinuclear factor, antiperinuclear factor), rheumatoid factors, immunoglobulins, and others [13]. Significantly increased circulating immune complexes were found in patients with Ménière's disease by Brookes [18] and Derebery et al. [19] and in patients with steroid-responsive sensorineural hearing loss by Kanzaki and O-Uchi [20].

Patient Population

At the Cleveland Clinic Foundation over the last 10 years, 101 patients were diagnosed; however, 54 returned to the care of referring physicians and follow-up audiometry was not available to report treatment results. The remaining 47 patients have been published previously [6] and are reviewed briefly here. Forty-four patients had positive LTT results. In 3 patients with Cogan's syndrome, test results were negative in 2 (presumably because the disease was not active) and not obtained in 1. Overall, the patient:control test ratio was 2.5 (normal < 1.7) with a range of 0.9 (false-negative result) to 4.8.

Twenty-nine patients were female, 18 were male. The average age was 44 years (range 6–76) at initial evaluation. Thirty-eight (81%) patients had bilateral disease and 9 unilateral. The presenting diagnosis consisted of four patterns: endolymphatic hydrops (Ménière's disease) (57%); progressive sensorineural hearing loss (22%); Cogan's syndrome (15%), and Dandy's syndrome (bilateral absent vestibular function with normal hearing) (6%). Sensorineural hearing loss, the hallmark of immune inner ear disease, was present in 94% of patients, usually rapidly progressive over a period of days or weeks. Thirteen patients (28%) had systemic immune disease: Cogan's syndrome (7), rheumatoid arthritis (3), temporal arteritis (1), Hashimoto's thyroiditis (1), or systemic vasculitits (1).

Low salt diet and diuretic were given for hydrops. The diuretic consisted usually of one capsule hydrochlorothiazide-triamterene daily. The initial steroid dose was prednisone 1 mg/kg/day. Some patients received high dose steroids only for 10 days in our early experience, but the majority received high doses for 30 days. Adult maintenance therapy consisted of prednisone 10 mg every other day for weeks or months, depending on the disease process, treatment response and drug tolerance. Cytotoxic drugs consisted of cyclophosphamide or nitrogen mustard in adults or methotrexate in children, usually for a 1-month trial. Lymphocytoplasmapheresis consisted of six treatments over 2 weeks. Thirty-seven patients received steroids, 34 low salt diet, 33 diuretics, 16 vestibular suppressants, 4 cytotoxic drugs, and 1 lymphocytoplasmapheresis. Most patients were treated with a combination of low salt diet, diuretic and steroid.

The pure tone average (500, 1,000 and 2,000 Hz) and word discrimination score were determined for both ears. The best pretreatment audiogram was compared with the most recent (i.e. longest posttreatment) audiogram. A significant difference was defined as greater than 10 dB pure tone average or 15% word discrimination score. Subjective change of dizziness was noted.

Follow-up averaged 2 years (range 1 month to 9 years). Hearing improved in at least one ear in 40% of patients, stabilized in at least one ear in 40%, and decreased in 20%. We consider stability of hearing a beneficial response when hearing was decreasing previously. Although the natural history of untreated disease is not known, apparently 80% of patients benefited from treatment within this limited follow-up period.

Furthermore, subjective symptoms of dizziness, fluctuating hearing, aural pressure and tinnitus improved in most patients and were not worse in any patient.

Discussion

Is autoimmune inner ear disease fact or fantasy? We believe it is a fact which will soon be proved; however, only immune-mediated disease thus far has been confirmed. Numerous studies (this article includes only a partial list of references) of antigen-specific humoral [3, 4, 10–12, 16], antigen-specific cellular [5, 6], and antigen-nonspecific [13, 14, 18–20] pathways strongly suggest that autoimmunity itself produces immune inner ear disease. We believe that clinical manifestations are relatively distinct, laboratory diagnosis is valid, and treatment is beneficial.

Most patients present with unexplained, rapidly progressive (weeks or months), bilateral sensorineural hearing loss. History, examination and radiographic studies help distinguish these patients from others with presbycusis, acoustic trauma, ototoxicity, infection, tumor and hereditary loss. Many patients have evidence for systemic immune disease, which suggests that immune ear disease can be primary or secondary. Some patients have symptoms of hydrops (Ménière's disease), which may be a nonspecific response to injury. In our experience, the patient at highest risk is middle-aged, often female, with bilateral progressive loss and systemic immune disease such as rheumatoid arthritis [21].

Antigen-specific tests, by definition, are more specific than antigen-nonspecific tests; therefore, they are preferred. No study has compared prospectively the predictive value of antigen-specific tests. We do not know why some investigators have had little or no success using the LTT [10, 17]; however, a great deal of time within our clinical laboratory is devoted to quality control of extracts. Perhaps our relative success stems from nearly 20 years of laboratory experience with the LTT as a diagnostic tool, for example, in beryllium lung disease [22]. The clinician always should interpret laboratory tests in light of the total clinical picture.

What are the sensitivity and specificity of the LTT? Sensitivity is the percent of true positive results when disease is present. LTT sensitivity is not known because it has not been measured prospectively [23]. In this retrospective review, 44 of 47 patients (94%) had positive results; however, when a positive result is used to confirm a presumptive diagnosis, retrospective measures of sensitivity will be artificially high. A prospective study of patients with Cogan's syndrome (ocular inflammation serves as a physical marker) would be more valid, when symptoms are active and the patient is not taking steroids. Unfortunately, Cogan's syndrome in our institution is so rare that a meaningful study would require many years. We estimate arbitrarily that test sensitivity is 70–80%.

Specificity is the percent of true negative results when disease is absent. Three separate studies of normal hospital volunteers have determined that LTT specificity is at least 93%. Of course, prospective testing of *otologic* controls would be better, but 93% probably is a valid estimate.

Calculation of the predictive value of a positive result requires not only test sensitivity and specificity but also disease prevalence. Again, disease prevalence is not known. However, if a test is sufficiently powerful (high sensitivity and specificity), a positive result can be used to estimate disease prevalence within a defined patient population. In a 2-year prospective study [23], all dizzy patients with bilateral *asymmetric* sensorineural hearing loss (to exclude presbycusis and similar problems), or with unilateral sensorineural hearing loss, were tested. The LTT was positive in 15%. These patients had negative radiographic and serologic studies to rule out tumor and syphilis.

If one estimates that disease prevalence is 15%, test sensitivity is 94% and specificity 93%, the predictive value of a positive LTT *in a suspect patient* is approximately 70% [23]. That is, 70% of positive results are true positives, and a positive result in a high risk patient should be interpreted as a true positive. A predictive value of 70% at first may seem artificially high, particularly when sensitivity is retrospectively estimated to be 94%. However, if specificity were 93% and prevalence 15%, sensitivities of 80 and 70% still would yield predictive values of 67 and 64% respectively, more than chance alone. Furthermore, if a study population consisted only of middle-aged women with bilateral Ménière's disease and rheumatoid arthritis, prevalence would be much higher. For example, if prevalence were 50%, sensitivity 94% and specificity 93%, the predictive value would rise to 93%.

No matter how the data are manipulated, the predictive value of a positive LTT in a suspect patient is greater than chance alone. Clinical manifestations and treatment results further support the validity of the test. The clinician should remember that false-negative results can occur if the disease is inactive or if the patient is taking immunosuppressant medication. If laboratory testing is not possible, a trial of steroids (we give prednisone 1 mg/kg/day for 1 month) should be given if there are no contraindications. No study has shown that steroid benefit is disease-specific; however, an 80% response rate in our patients (40% improved and 40% stabilized with an average 2-year-follow-up) supports both the diagnosis and the validity of the LTT.

The major drawback to the LTT is that it is not widely available. However, in North America a sample of whole fresh blood can be mailed to our regional laboratory by overnight carrier [21], and the results are known in approximately 7 days. The test costs approximately $120. Better tests will be developed when the putative antigens are discovered; however, for now we remain very pleased with the LTT in the laboratory diagnosis of immune inner ear disease.

Conclusions

(1) Relatively distinct clinical manifestations, valid laboratory testing, and beneficial treatment response in patients, and experimental studies in animals, indicate clearly that immune-mediated inner ear disease is a fact.

(2) Autoimmune inner ear disease no longer is fantasy, and will be confirmed soon.

References

1 Lehnhardt E: Plötzliche Hörstörungen, auf beiden Seiten gleichzeitig oder nacheinander aufgetreten. Z Laryngol Rhinol Otol 1958;37:1.
2 Kikuchi M: On the 'sympathetic otitis'. Zibi Rinsyo Kyoto 1959;52:600.
3 Beichert P: Zur Frage der Empfindungsschwerhörigkeit und Autoallergie. Z Laryngol Rhinol Otol 1961;40:837.
4 Terayama Y, Yukihiro S: Studies on experimental allergic (isoimmune) labyrinthitis in guinea pigs. Acta otolaryngol (Stockh) 1963;58:49–64.
5 McCabe BF: Autoimmune sensorineural hearing loss. Ann Otol Rhinol Laryngol 1979;88:585–589.
6 Hughes GB, Barna BP, Kinney SE, et al: Immune inner ear disease: 1990 report. Ann Otol Rhinol Laryngol, in press.
7 Oppenheim JJ, Shecter B: Lymphocyte transformation; in Manual of Clinical Immunology, ed 2. Washington, American Society of Microbiology, 1980, pp 233–245.
8 Hughes GB, Kinney SE, Barna BP, et al: Autoimmune reactivity in Ménière's disease: preliminary report. Laryngoscope 1983;43:410–417.

9   Rockline RE: Production and assay of macrophage inhibitory factor; in Manual of Clinical Immunology, ed 2. Washington, American Society of Microbiology, 1980, pp 246–251.

10   Arnold W, Pfaltz CR, Altermatt HJ: Evidence of serum antibodies against inner ear tissues in the blood of patients with certain sensorineural disorders. Acta Otolaryngol (Stockh) 1985;99:437.

11   Arnold W, Pfaltz CR: Critical evaluation of the immunofluorescence. A microscopic test for identification of serum antibodies against human inner ear tissue. Acta Otolaryngol (Stockh) 1987;103:373–378.

12   Soliman AM: Optimizing immunofluorescence for the testing of autoantibodies in inner ear disorders. Arch Otolaryngol 1988;245:28–35.

13   Veldman JE: Immune-mediated inner ear disorders: New syndromes and their etiopathogenesis; in Veldman JE, McCabe BF (eds): Oto-Immunology. Amsterdam, Kugler, 1987, pp 125–141.

14   Elies W, Plester D: Immunological findings in various sensorineural hearing disorders; in Veldman JE, McCabe BF (eds): Oto-Immunology. Amsterdam, Kugler, 1987, pp 157–161.

15   Gosslau B, Barrach HJ: Enzyme-linked immunosorbent microassay for quantification of specific antibodies to collagen type I, II, III. J Immunol Methods 1979;29: 71–77.

16   Orozco CR, Niparko JK, Richardson BC, et al: Experimental model of immune-mediated hearing loss employing cross-species immunization. Laryngoscope, in press.

17   Harris JP, Sharp PA: Inner ear autoantibodies in patients with rapidly progressive sensorineural hearing loss. Laryngoscope 1990;100:516–524.

18   Brookes GB: Circulating immune complexes in Ménière's disease. J Laryngol Otol 1986;100:21–24.

19   Derebery MJ, Rao A, Siglock T, et al: Circulating immune complexes in Ménière's disease. Laryngoscope, in press.

20   Kanzaki J, O-Uchi T: Circulating immune complexes in steroid responsive sensorineural hearing loss and the long-term observation. Acta Otolaryngol (Stockh) 1983 (suppl 393):77–84.

21   Hughes GB, Barna BP, Kinney SE, et al: Clinical diagnosis of immune inner ear disease. Laryngoscope 1988;48:251–253.

22   Deodar SD, Barna BP, Van Orstrand HS: A study of the immunologic aspects of chronic berylliosis. Chest 1973;63:309–313.

23   Hughes GB, Barna BP, Kinney SE, et al: Predictive value of laboratory tests in autoimmune inner ear disease. Laryngoscope 1986;96:502–505.

Gordon B. Hughes, MD, Department of Otolaryngology and Communicative Disorders, A–1, One Clinic Center, Cleveland, OH 44195 (USA)

Pfaltz CR, Arnold W, Kleinsasser O (eds): Bearing of Basic Research on Clinical Otolaryngology. Adv Otorhinolaryngol. Basel, Karger, 1991, vol 46, pp 92–96

Discussion

Arnold (Luzern): I think it is important to make the difference whether the antigen, which is involved in the immunopathological process, is localized within the inner ear or not. Let us take the best candidate – to me it's the hair cell. This is a highly specialized cell and I suspect that it must have specialized molecules, perhaps on the surface; and if these molecules would be hit by antibodies one would have a true autoimmune disease of the inner ear. In this condition I doubt that it will be a bilateral disease but assume it would be unilateral. However, an antigen which is systemic might be distributed to both organs. I can imagine that in this instance a unilateral disposition may occur in case the inner ear vessels have perhaps some primary lesion which causes a locus of minor resistance. Dr. Schuknecht, did you always find the described alterations or pathology? You collected some temporal bones from patients affected with a well-known and well-described systemic autoimmune disease? Could you always find typical alterations in both ears?

Schuknecht (Boston): Yes – I neglected to mention that, but the changes were almost identical in the two ears. The only two differences were that one ear had a Cody-tac in it and the other difference was that one ear had a blocked vestibular aqueduct. I think it is important to point out also that the cochlear neurons were normal in both ears which rules out the possibility that these changes could have been induced by a vascular lesion, because in animals if you block the vascular supply so that it affects both the cochlear and vestibular systems like in this ear then you always get severe degeneration of the cochlear neurons.

Arnold: But the pathological type of reaction, is that one of an inflammation and the consequence of it?

Schuknecht: No. This is a real inflammatory lesion that we are looking at here in this patient. Of course in the animals where you block the vascular supply we do not have an inflammatory lesion such as this, you have an ischemic necrosis and then the build up of fibrous tissue and new bone formation.

Arnold: A question to Dr. Harris: Is there evidence which supports the involvement of primary autonomy in certain types of inner ear disorders or what is the evidence against it, what do you think?

Harris (San Diego): Are you speaking of isolated organs?

Arnold: I mean is there some evidence as you could show in your experiments that this possibility exists in humans too, or how would you translate your experimental findings into the clinical symptomatology?

Harris: The only evidence that we have currently – circumstantial evidence as we heard before, is not conclusive because if you are looking at the antibody in the serum that does not necessarily represent the etiology in the inner ear and could be the consequence of damage to the ear in release of an antigen subsequently of exposure or what we may call an epiphenomenon. So it may not be necessarily the etiology of the disease but it may be important diagnostically as a marker for the disease. I do not think that there is specific evidence.

Arnold: Most of the members of the auditorium are clinicians, so they are interested in diagnostic procedures and on therapy. Dr. Veldman, what is the best diagnostic test battery available at the present time? What would you recommend to do if there is a patient who is suspect of having an immunomediated disease of the ear? Do you select your patients before testing the antibody – that means do you test only certain patients where you have some information that they could have an immunomediated inner ear disease and what is the basis of this selection?

Veldman (Utrecht): Let me start with laboratory tests which have no standard to the general population. If you get more positives than two positives so you must apply to clinically suspicious patients. The patient in our practice who is at highest risk is a middle-aged patient, often a woman with bilateral progressive sensorineural hearing loss not otherwise to explain, with or without dizziness, who may also have some evidence for a systemic immune problem. When I have a suspicious patient whose symptoms are active and who is not taking cortisone or other immunosuppressive medication I will give a trial of high dose prednisone for 1 month if there are no contraindications. Then I repeat the hearing test. And the corroboration of the clinical exams, laboratory tests and the treatment with drugs help me to reach a probable diagnosis.

Arnold: Will you also treat a patient who has a negative test result but a clinical picture which gives you the feeling that this must be an immunomediated disease?

Veldman: Very often, patients are referred to me for a second opinion who are on some type of lower steroid treatment. Then I am so concerned that I might be getting a false-negative lab test that I will instead bump the patient on to a high dose for 1 month and after that the patient comes off steroids at some future date. If symptoms recur at that time I would try to get a lab test for confirmation. So the answer to your question is yes. I give steroids hoping that they may help to improve the hearing.

Arnold: How will you treat a patient with slowly progressive sensorineural hearing loss who is otherwise healthy and who has no family history?

Veldman: I think you have to divide this problem. First of all I describe the easy cases because they have a systemic autoimmune disease, they are clinically and immunologically positive and they get hearing symptoms. We do not treat them aggressively but we are solid in our conception that we should treat them with steroids. I think that is no question. The problem is also not that particular group. You see, to give an example: An only one-hearing-ear patient comes in with a heavily progressive hearing loss, you find a sensorineuronal hearing loss with or without vestibular symptoms, you have a feeling that he may belong to that particular group of say 'autoimmune inner ear disease'. Even if no systemical clinical positive test in that particular patient is present, he should be treated. Give him a trial and just wait and see whether the ear drys up. I think everybody would go for it and treat it. The real problem is the middle group – the slowly progressive sensori-neuronal hearing loss, which looks a little bit like Ménière's disease maybe yes, maybe no. How do you treat him? That is very questionable. If the tests are negative, should you give steroids and even go up to sudden toxicity, yes or no? I don't think so.

Arnold: I've got a question for Dr. Harris: You mentioned that autoimmune inner ear disease has not been proven yet, but what is your present philosophy concerning this unproven disease?

Harris: The case that I presented had evidence of continuous lesions, febrile course, pain in the ears and you saw the audiometric profiles and vestibular profiles plus the fact that the histopathology looks very similar to those cases where you have systemic autoimmune disease. Very similar, plus the fact that there is no other disease that I have ever seen in temporal bones. It looks like this. This is something different, something new. I have never seen this kind of pathology before. So I think the evidence is building up very strongly. I know that you would like postulates confirming that, but I think it's time to be moving off face a little bit.

Arnold: But we don't have a test to prove that there is an isolated autoimmune inner ear disease. So at the moment, if I would write a textbook or you would write a textbook, would you use the terminus *autoimmune disease of the inner ear?*

Harris: I think I would.

Arnold: I still hesitate to do that – I would write probably *immunomediated disease* or disease of the inner ear as a part of an autoimmune disease.

Harris: I'm known to be a sceptic. But I am so strongly convinced about this, it's going to appear in my revision of 'Pathology of the Inner Ear' as a specific disease entity. I would not consider this a battle. I'm only suggesting that when you have a patient with systemic symptoms of immunological problems such as eosinophilia, febrile illness, that's suggested that there is a systemic problem, a systemic autoimmune disease. This partic-ular patient I mentioned also had audiovestibular symptoms. The distinction that we are trying to make is that there are patients without any systemic symptoms, without any evidence of autoimmune disease in their body except for the inner ear and it is that only distinction I'm trying to make. I still think that when you have a patient whose audio-vestibular symptoms are so dominant for so many years – in this case approximately from 1983 to 1986 audiovestibular symptoms were a predominant problem – the other symp-toms are smiled at and minimal by comparison. I would think that you would be justified in calling that an inner ear problem.

Arnold: Dr. Melchers you know I do not want that we only change from the term 'idiopathic' to the term 'autoimmune' because that does not give us anything. So to make the definite diagnosis of an autoimmune disease of the inner ear I think it is absolutely necessary to have a reliable test which we do not have. The pathologist is in the advantage that he sits 8 or 10 years later at the microscope seeing the results and he can build up the whole story from the history of the patient. He concludes that this must be a typical case because he knows that the patient has suffered from a systemic autoimmune disease. But there are also temporal bones where you only have proliferation of tissue and ossification which could be the consequence of a mild unspecific inflammation or I don't know what. Is a specific test in fact necessary to use the terminus 'autoimmune' inner ear disease?

Melchers (Basel): I think I would like to warn of getting too far into semantics. I think what's behind is far more important. I think everybody would agree that after what we have heard from Dr. Harris that at least there are cases in which you can induce a normal immune response in the inner ear and that immune response you wonder sometimes why that exists. The second you can ask is, if there is an immune response occurring in the inner ear that can be diverged to become pathological then, of course, there must be or there could be infectious agents. That initiates the inner ear disease. Then it would become pathological just as much as some virus infection in the brain that you could call autoimmune, because it destroys its own tissues. But there is a certain antigen that comes from the outside, so my suspicion would be that first of all the ordinary disease is at the beginning of the inner ear lesion. We do not know that yet exactly and every pathological effect we see later can either be due to an inside or an outside antigen. I would not dismiss at the moment either one of the 2 cases and it would be certainly safe to call it 'immune'.

Arnold: Why I insist in this question is, we want to treat our patients and we want to give a rational basis of the treatment for example with cortisone or cytotoxic drugs. And if we are doing that we must have some idea what is happening within the ear. The simple question I always put is: If your son, otherwise a completely healthy person, would have a bilateral sensorineural hearing loss, and the hearing loss increases from month to month, and you have no indication of an autoimmune disease, would you treat him with high dosages of cortisone or endoxan – yes or no? That is also a question to the panel because we have to answer it every day.

Harris: Well, the contraindications to steroids are well known and assuming that there are no contraindications, I see no reason to withhold the trial of steroids, they may help and whether you can prove it's an autoimmune phenomenon who cares – the patient does not want to go deaf and that's the bottom line.

Arnold: Thank you, this answer makes me very happy. Dr. Veldman – What do you think about this problem?

Veldman: That's a similar example as the only hearing ear; of course, I think I'll go for it in a case like that. The problem for the audience is particularly the problem of those who are somewhere in the middle: Do they belong to the group, yes or no? We will give them a trial treatment.

Arnold: Are we able to make a recommendation of the dosage and of the duration of the treatment?

Veldman: The way this is done in our department is the following: When we are dealing with systemic autoimmune diseases with an expression in the inner ear, our experience is that we treat them with 2 mg prednisone per kilogram body weight up to a maximum of about 80 or 100 mg/day. And I treat them for about 2 weeks and see what happens. Our experience is in those cases that they will respond very heavily or they don't respond, then we will take them off. In the case in which the son of the doctor has only one single functioning ear we may add endoxan 2 mg/kg body weight orally a similar period of time. If he does not respond, we will question ourselves again what we should do. But then we have to be very cautious in each individual case we are dealing with. With one hearing ear we will go on. If both ears are involved, but not so heavily, I think we will stop because we feel there is no effect. At any rate we are not going on for 3-month trials.

Arnold: Are there any questions from the auditory?

Shambaugh (Hinsdale): This was a perfectly marvellous group of papers and enormously stimulating. I am very interested in zinc. Zinc is the only nutriate that the thymus gland must have to function normally and I was very impressed by the first speaker who mentioned how the thymus gland must function in order to process the lymphatic cells properly and to protect the autoimmunity. I myself have had a sudden deafness in one ear. Two attacks. The last attack was a total deafness, absolutely no response at all. Recovered with prednisone 60 mg/day for 2 weeks. I'm sure I had this syndrome. I'm allergic since childhood; I can bring this on by overindulging in this antigen.

Arnold: Why don't we have more temporal bones from patients with so-called autoimmune diseases?

Schuknecht: It is a rather rare disorder compared to, for example, Ménière's disease, sudden deafness, otosclerosis, presbycusis; you can go on and on and, therefore, this is the only case that I have been able to acquire and this came too through the temporal bone bank. The only ears that look very similar to this one I showed you today are those ears from patients who develop deafness from measles and those are usually bilateral like this but the difference is clinically, i.e. the hearing loss as such. In this patient we could possibly do with measles. To me this is a very special case because that's a different disorder that I have never seen before and it's unique. I believe it to be autoimmune without any question.

Burian (Wien): If there is a patient successfully treated with cortisone, what happens after finishing this treatment, if you assume there is an autoimmune disease? Would you expect a final recurrence after a short time?

Veldman: The treatment is stopped in those say not so heavy cases of systemic autoimmunity; you can stop the treatment and they are not drug dependent with respect to the hearing loss. However, you may find other cases if you are aware of them; I recall one of the cases we have seen, an older lady who comes to the rheumatologist and to our department when her rheumatory arthritis is active and she gets steroids from her internist; she puts the hearing aid in deposit when the rheumatory arthritis goes down clinically and the steroids are not necessary anymore. After that her hearing goes down again and she comes back to the hearing aids. So some seem to be low dose prednisone dependent. I think other people have made similar experiences.

Arnold: Thank you very much. Is there any important additional question from the auditorium or somebody who could give some additional information? If not, I will finish this morning's session with a very simple summary. And this summary is my personal opinion: That means that we have to deal with immunomediated inner ear diseases which are as far as we know part of a systemic immunological process. This would justify to treat an inner ear hearing loss under this condition with immunosuppressive substances. But at the moment, I personally am not convinced that we have the right to speak about an isolated autoimmune disease of the inner ear yet. Please excuse me if somebody of the panel has a different opinion, but we don't have all the scientific proof necessary to create and to teach such a term. Thank you for listening.

Epidemiology, Etiology and Pathogenesis of Head and Neck Cancer

Introduction

In spite of improved diagnosing and progresses in therapy we have to note a continuously increasing incidence of malignant tumours. In addition to the well-known carcinogens for the upper aerodigestive tract like alcohol and tobacco, more and more other influences such as virus infections, pollution or occupational exposures are believed to cause malignant tumours of the head and neck. In the FRG for example the number of tumours recognized as occupational diseases had a fivefold increase from 1978 to 1988.

The only chance to reduce the incidence of head and neck cancers consists in improving prevention. People should be made aware of the well-known carcinogens such as tobacco and alcohol. The hitherto unknown carcinogens have to be discovered and eliminated. Therefore a good cooperation between clinicians and epidemiologists is of great importance. While the clinician makes some observations and supposes that the tumour might be connected with external influences, the epidemiologist uses statistical methods and whatever data is available to prove the suspicion. A very good example of this is the discovery of wood dust as a carcinogen for sinonasal cancer. The clinical otorhinolaryngologists Hadfield and Macbeth observed that many joiners were taken ill with nasal adenocarcinoma. This observation was then substantiated by the studies of the epidemiologist Acheson, who found an enormously elevated risk for this occupational group to get nasal adenocarcinoma.

To develop programs in cancer prevention and to reduce risks related to occupational or environmental carcinogens we have to engage in epidemiology, aetiology and pathogenesis of malignant tumours. In the following papers, qualified authors will comment on this subject and expound the present situation of scientific findings.

H.-G. Schroeder

Pfaltz CR, Arnold W, Kleinsasser O (eds): Bearing of Basic Research on Clinical
Otolaryngology. Adv Otorhinolaryngol. Basel, Karger, 1991, vol 46, pp 98–106

Aetiology of Head and Neck Cancer:
Tobacco, Alcohol and Diet

A.J. Tuyns

Unit of Analytical Epidemiology, IARC, Lyon, France

This paper deals with cancer of larynx and hypopharynx, mouth and oesophagus. The aetiology of tumours of nasal cavities and nasopharynx is essentially different and is dealt with in other sections of this book.

Our knowledge of the aetiology of laryngeal, hypopharyngeal and oral cancer rests on clinical and epidemiological observations. These are dominated by three features, namely: (a) the predominance of these tumours among males; (b) their unusual geographic distribution, and (c) changes of incidence with time.

The *predominance* of laryngeal cancer *in males* and its relative rarity in females is a common clinical observation. It is corroborated by very high sex ratios ranging from 2 to 20 and more.

The *geographic distribution* of laryngeal cancer in Europe is illustrated in figure 1. The highest mortality rates are observed in France, Spain and Italy, while the rates are much lower in the other countries. This distribution is of particular interest insofar as it is in sharp contrast with the distribution of lung cancer [1] (fig. 2). Within Switzerland, the highest rates are noted in the 'cantons' of the West and South [2].

Increase with time: In Denmark and in Connecticut, USA, cancer registries have been in operation for several decades; incidence data are available for analyses of time trends. There is a definite increase of incidence over time but not so important as for lung cancer [1] (fig. 3, 4). It is of interest to note that this increase of the incidence is more marked than a more moderate increase in mortality.

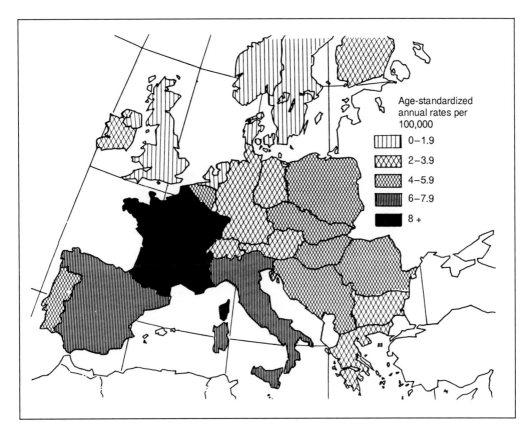

Fig. 1. Cancer of larynx mortality in males, 1975–1976.

Tobacco: All the features described above are consistent with the role of tobacco, which has been identified for a long time. It has been confirmed and analysed ever since large prospective studies were set up for studying the effects of smoking. The two main American studies, the study on British doctors and the large Japanese study all showed mortality ratios ranging from 6 to 13 [3]. Other studies showed an increase of risk with amount smoked and with duration of smoking; also, with filter cigarettes, the risk is slightly lower than with nonfilters [4].

Even though there is no doubt as to the deleterious effect of smoking, the tobacco hypothesis cannot explain the contrast observed in Europe between the south-west countries and the rest of the continent. Why should

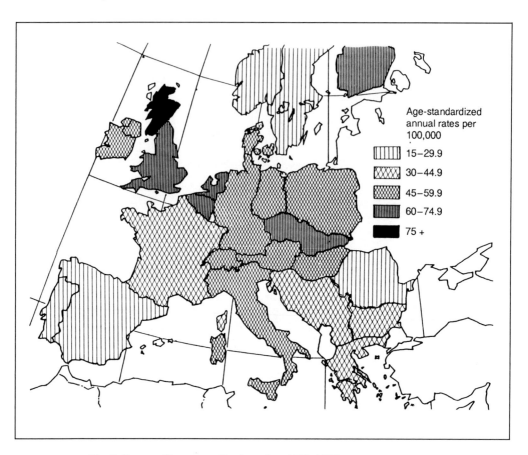

Fig. 2. Cancer of lung mortality in males, 1975–1976.

smoking increase lung cancer rates in the United Kingdom and in the Benelux countries and increase laryngeal cancers in France, Italy and Spain? Additional hypotheses are needed to explain this contrast. Some relate to type of tobacco. In Latin countries, smokers use dark air-cured tobacco, while in most other countries people prefer the 'light' flue-cured tobacco (blond). The latter has been shown to be less aggressive and less carcinogenic [5]. Thus, one could imagine that dark tobacco reaching the larynx would induce cancer in that organ, while light tobacco smoke could penetrate deeper in the respiratory tract and then induce lung cancer.

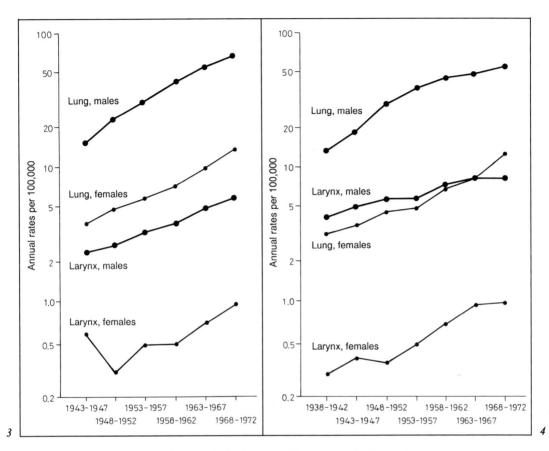

Fig. 3. Incidence time trends for larynx and lung cancer in Denmark.
Fig. 4. Incidence time trends for larynx and lung cancer in Connecticut.

Alcohol: There are however alternative hypotheses, and exposures other than tobacco need to be considered. In the south-west of Europe the consumption of alcoholic beverages – particularly of wine – is important; alcohol could be suspected to be a risk factor. In fact, the national mortality figures for laryngeal cancer correlate better with average alcohol intake than with tobacco consumption [1] (fig. 5). Furthermore, there is good evidence for cancer of the mouth [6] and for cancer of the oesophagus [7] that alcohol and tobacco combine their effects according to a model compatible with a multiplicative effect.

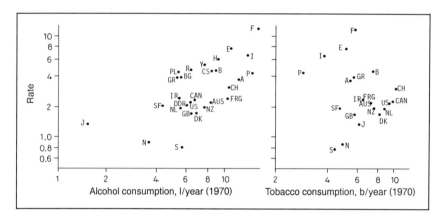

Fig. 5. Laryngeal cancer mortality: age-standardized annual rates per 100,000 males, 1975–1976. Correlation with alcohol consumption and with tobacco consumption.

It was logical to think that alcohol might be related to laryngeal cancer as well. This was by no means a new hypothesis. Clinicians were used to notice that their patients were very often heavy drinkers as well as heavy smokers. In their case-control studies carried out in New York, Wynder et al. [4] had shown a combination of effects of tobacco and alcohol, the latter operating among heavy smokers.

More recent studies in Canada [8, 9] suggested that alcohol might play a more important role than hitherto believed. Yet all these studies were carried out in populations with a rather moderate consumption of alcohol, i.e. in comparison with countries like France, Italy or Spain, where an average daily intake of 500 to 1,000 ml of wine is not uncommon in males. Hence the idea of undertaking an epidemiological investigation in the latter countries, to test the hypotheses mentioned above, as well as additional factors such as diet and professional exposures.

The IARC Study on Laryngeal and Hypopharyngeal Cancer in South-West Europe

The places selected for the study were Torino and Varese in Italy, Zaragoza and Pamplona in Spain, and the Département of Calvados (where previous studies on oesophageal cancer had been carried out);

Table 1. Modification of risk with various parameters relating to smoking

		Endolarynx	Hypopharynx/epilarynx
Average cigarette consumption	0	1	1
	1–7	2.37	4.18
	8–15	6.68	10.79
	16–25	13.69	15.80
	26+	16.42	16.11
	ever smoked	9.91	12.37
Years since quitting	current smokers	1	1
	1–4	1.51	1.09
	5–9	0.52	0.28
	10+	0.28	0.32
Use of filter	only plain	1	1
	only filter	0.49	0.47
Type of tobacco	only blond	1	1
	only black	1.98	2.16
Inhalation	inhalers	1	1
	noninhalers	0.66	0.87

Geneva joined in the endeavour. In all these places there was a good cancer registration system, permitting a fairly good coverage of all cases occurring during the investigation.

Various problems relating to the exact location of the tumour had to be solved and are discussed in another section of this book by Prof. Lehmann, who was in charge of reviewing systematically all the clinical files contributed by the various study centres [10]. In this paper, the discussion will be limited to the analyses concerning the role of tobacco and alcohol [11].

The findings on tobacco are summarized in table 1. One of the main findings concerned the amount smoked daily: the risk increases rapidly and considerably with number of cigarettes per day, as well for endolarynx as for hypopharynx and epilarynx. For those who stopped smoking, the risk decreases with time and is reduced by some 70% after 10 years.

Table 2. Risks related to alcohol consumption

Average daily consumption of alcohol, g/day	Endolarynx	Hypopharynx/epilarynx
0–20	1	1
21–40	0.94	1.23
41–80	1.06	2.43
81–120	1.71	5.19
121+	2.56	11.37

The risk of users of filter cigarettes was about half the risk of those smoking cigarettes without filters. All these findings confirmed those of Wynder et al. [4] and other authors [8, 9]. In addition, it was found that smokers of dark tobacco have about twice the risk of those smoking 'blond' tobacco. The role of inhalation, known to be of importance for lung cancer, was also examined. It increases slightly the risk of cancer of the endolarynx but has practically no effect for cancer of the hypopharynx and epilarynx.

As to the role of alcohol (table 2), it is present in both groups; it is particularly important for hypopharynx and epilarynx. Interestingly, in the large number of cases under study (more than a thousand), only 34 smokers were non-drinkers; there were also 31 lifetime nonsmokers all of whom were drinkers.

The combined role of tobacco and alcohol was analysed in the same way as was done previously for cancer of the mouth [6] and cancer of the oesophagus [7]. In both groups of tumours, the two factors are multiplicative (fig. 6). For hypopharynx and epilarynx the role of alcohol predominates; for endolarynx the effect of tobacco seems to be more important than the role of alcohol. This difference makes sense, considering the differential exposure to tobacco smoke and to alcoholic beverages in the two anatomical locations.

The analyses have not yet been completed on the role of diet. There is, however, an indication of a protective role of ascorbic acid. As to professional exposures, the investigations are still under way. There seems to be an effect of exposure to asbestos – an effect described by other authors.

In terms of *practical implications* and of *prevention,* things are clear: both tobacco and alcohol are the main causal factors of laryngeal and

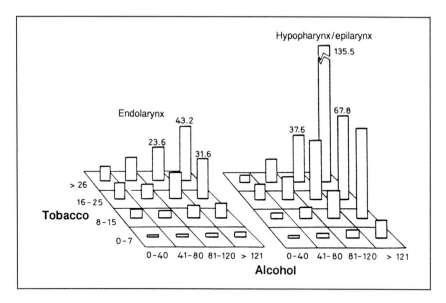

Fig. 6. Relative risks according to daily consumption of tobacco and alcohol (g/day).

hypopharyngeal cancer. Reducing – if not quitting – consumption of tobacco and of alcohol would result in a considerable decrease of incidence of these cancers.

References

1   Tuyns, A.J.: Incidence trends of laryngeal cancer in relation to national alcohol and tobacco consumption; in Magnus, K. (ed): Trends in cancer incidence, causes and practical implications, pp. 199–214 (Hemisphere, Washington 1982).
2   Office Fédéral de la Statistique: La distribution géographique de la mortalité cancéreuse en Suisse, 1979/1981 (Office Fédéral de la Statistique, Berne 1984).
3   US Department of Health, Education and Welfare: Smoking and health. A report of the Surgeon General. DHEW Publ. No. (PHS) 79–50066 (1979).
4   Wynder, E.L.; Covey, L.S.; Mabouchi, K.; Mushinski, M.: Environmental factors in cancer of the larynx. A second look. Cancer *38:* 1591–1601 (1976).
5   Benhamou, S.; Benhamou, E.; Tirmarche, M.; Flamant, R.: Lung cancer and use of cigarettes. A French case-control study. J. natl. Cancer Inst. *74:* 1169–1175 (1985).

6   Rothman, K.J.; Keller, A.: The effect of joint exposure to alcohol and tobacco on risk of cancer of the mouth and pharynx. J. chron. Dis. *25:* 711–716 (1972).

7   Tuyns, A.J.; Pequignot, G.; Jensen, O.M.: Le cancer de l'œsophage en Ille et Vilaine en fonction des niveaux de consommation d'alcool et de tabac. Des risques qui se multiplient. Bull. Cancer *64:* 45–60 (1977).

8   Birch, J.D.; Howe, G.R.; Miller, A.B.; Semenciw, R.: Tobacco, alcohol, asbestos and nickel in the etiology of cancer of the larynx: a case-control study. J. natl. Cancer Inst. *67:* 1219–1224 (1981).

9   Elwood, J.M.; Pearson, J.C.G.; Skippen, D.H.; Jackson, S.M.: Alcohol, smoking and occupational factors in the aetiology of cancer of the oral cavity, pharynx and larynx. Int. J Cancer *34:* 603–612 (1984).

10 Lehmann, W.; Raymond, L.; Blanchet, F.; Sancho-Garnier, H.; Pequignot, G.; Estève, J.; Tuyns, A.J.: Epidémiologie et étiologie spécifique des cancers du larnyx et de l'hypopharynx en Europe du sud-ouest; in Kellerhals, B., et al.: ORL 11 Problèmes actuels d'Otorhinolaryngologie (Huber, Bern 1988).

11 Tuyns, A.J.; Estève, J.; Raymond, L.; Berrino, F.; Benhamou, E.; Blanchet, F.; Boffetta, P.; Crosignani, P.; Del Moral, A.; Lehmann, W.; Merletti, F.; Pequignot, G.; Riboli, E.; Sancho-Garnier, H.; Terracini, B.; Zubiri, A.; Zubiri, L.: Cancer of the larynx/hypopharynx, tobacco and alcohol. Int. J. Cancer *41:* 483–491 (1988).

Dr. A.J. Tuyns, Unit of Analytical Epidemiology, IARC,
150, cours A.-Thomas, F–69372 Lyon Cedex 08 (France)

Pfaltz CR, Arnold W, Kleinsasser O (eds): Bearing of Basic Research on Clinical Otolaryngology. Adv Otorhinolaryngol. Basel, Karger, 1991, vol 46, pp 107–115

Adenocarcinomas of the Nose after Exposure to Wood Dust

Heinz-Georg Schroeder

Ear-Nose-Throat Clinic, Philipps University, Marburg/Lahn, FRG

The first paper that suggested a causal connection between a chemical noxa and nasal cancer was published in 1761 by John Hill [1]. He accused 'the immoderate use of snuff' of being an important cause of nasal cancer. It nearly took 200 years till in the 20th century several other chemical substances or working processes were suspected to induce nasal cancer, e.g. nickel, chromates, isopropyl oils, asbestos, arsenic, mustard gas, tar smoke, inhalation of radioactive isotopes, shoe and textile manufacturing, and after all, woodworking. Not all of them are recognized as occupational cancers in the different countries.

During the last 12 years, 83 cases of nasal cancer have been accepted as occupational disease (table 1) [2]. Adenocarcinomas after wood dust exposure are by far the most frequent occupational nasal cancers in Ger-

Table 1. Nasal cancers accepted as occupational disease by the German Industrial Injuries Insurance Institute for the Woodworking Industry, 1978–1990

Noxa	Cases
Ionizing radiation	1
Nickel	1
Chromates	3
Tar, tar oils	6
Halogenized alkyloxide	1
Mineral oil	3
Wood dust	68 (82%)
	83

many. Nasal adenocarcinomas are rare tumours which had been published as case reports in the first half of our century. The occurrence of those tumours after wood dust exposure was first described by Macbeth and Hadfield [3] in 1965. This report from England has since been verified by a number of authors in various countries. In newer reviews of the literature more than 800 cases have been registered all over the world [4, 5]. It is a remarkable fact that only less than 10% of all cases have been published by non-European authors.

Materials and Methods

There have been no unequivocal indications concerning a direct correlation between tumour and wood dust in West Germany so far. In order to examine this condition the German Industrial Injuries Insurance Institute for the Woodworking Industry (Holz-Berufsgenossenschaft) tried to get information about all cases of adenocarcinoma in our country. All West German ENT clinics were requested to notify their cases; a total of 122 adenocarcinomas could be collected. In all cases we obtained detailed occupational histories [6]. In the Marburg ENT Clinic we studied the clinical histories and examined the original histological slides. We differentiated three main groups of adenocarcinoma (table 2) [5, 7].

The various adenocarcinomas of the mucous glands are in the first group, such as adenoid cystic carcinomas, mucoepidermoid tumours, acinic cell tumours and others. The second group consists of the so-called 'terminal tubulus adenocarcinomas'. This entity was first separated and described by Kleinsasser [8, 9] in 1984. Histogenetically this tumour originates from the nasal mucoserous glands and shows low grade malignancy. The tumours of the third group are histologically very similar to adenocarcinomas of the gastrointestinal tract. Therefore they are denoted as 'intestinal type' or 'colonic type' tumours. We could find strong correlation between wood dust exposure and tumour only

Table 2. Histological classification of nasal adenocarcinomas collected by the German Industrial Injuries Insurance Institute for the Woodworking Industry diagnosed 1948–1985 (notified 1979–1985)

	Cases	Wood dust exposure
Adenocarcinomas of the mucous glands (adenoic cystic carcinomas, mucoepidermoid tumours, acinic cell tumours, etc.)	27	1 (3.7%)
Terminal tubulus adenocarcinomas	18	2 (11.1%)
Intestinal type adenocarcinomas	77	67 (87.0%) ⎫ 123
additionally diagnosed 1985–1989		56 ⎭
	122	

in this group of adenocarcinomas. In the last 4 years another 56 cases of this tumour type have been notified so that we now survey 123 cases of intestinal type adenocarcinoma after wood dust exposure.

Morphology

As in gastrointestinal tumours, the intestinal type adenocarcinomas can be classified into different subtypes. The majority, 94 cases, are the 'papillary tubular cylindrical cell adenocarcinomas'. Fifteen cases in our series can be classified as 'alveolar mucinous goblet cell adenocarcinomas'. With 4 cases, the rarest form observed was the 'signet ring cell adenocarcinoma'. In addition to these pure types, 10 cases with transition from one type to another were found. Although being morphologically distinct, these transitional types give a clue to the close histogenetic relationship between the three subtypes.

The 'papillary tubular cylindrical cell adenocarcinoma' shows papillary and tubular formations side by side in the same tumour. The highly cylindrical tumour cells with basally lying nuclei form one layer of densely packed cells. The 'alveolar mucinous goblet cell adenocarcinoma' exhibits large glandular alveolar formations with abundant mucous secretion. Some of the cells are very similar to goblet cells. They produce so much mucus that the glandular tubes burst and float like garlands in the lake of mucus. Similar pictures can be seen in intestinal adenocarcinomas. All tumour cells of the 'signet ring cell adenocarcinoma' are completely filled with mucus. Only a few cells are connected to solid formations, most of the signet ring cells float in the lake of mucus. In all four types we found the same strong correlation to wood dust exposure. The various types of these adenocarcinomas all seem to originate from one parent cell, an apocrinous mucus-secreting cylinder cell. The different morphological appearances seem to correspond to various stages of development and function of this parent cell.

Epidemiological Data

Among the 123 cases of wood dust-induced nasal adenocarcinomas, there were only 2 female woodworkers. This may be explained by the fact that women in Germany by tradition had different tasks in wood processing with less dusty work places. The age of all cases ranges from 25 to 85

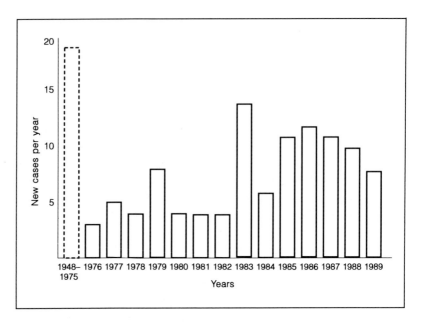

Fig. 1. New cases of nasal adenocarcinoma distributed to the years of their first diagnosis.

years with a median age of 56 years. If we distribute all cases to the years of their first diagnosis, it seems that we have to expect 10–15 new cases per year (fig. 1). It was only during the last 5 years that we could completely register all new tumours.

After evaluating the detailed occupational histories of the 123 persons with intestinal type adenocarcinoma we found that all had been exposed to oak or beech wood dust. No cases had been exposed exclusively to dust of soft or exotic woods. Wood dust concentrations at their work place were usually more than 10 mg/m³, in extreme cases up to 500 mg/m³. Most of them had been employed in small workshops, only a few in industrial wood work [6]. The 123 persons pursued 141 wood occupations. The majority worked as joiners or cabinet makers. But we also found several occupations which are nowadays rather rare, like cartwrights, coopers, builders of wooden shutters or orthopaedic shoemakers and others (table 3).

The duration of exposure ranged from 2 to 50 years with a median time of 32 years. The shortest duration of exposure we found in the literature was 18 months, reported from England [10]. The latency period var-

Table 3. Occupations of 123 persons with nasal adenocarcinoma after wood dust exposure

Occupation	Cases
Joiner/cabinet maker	93
Cartwright	14
Cooper	9
Parquet floor layer	5
Carpenter	5
Boat builder	3
Orthopaedic shoemaker	2
Shutter builder	2
Others	8

ied from 4 to 70 years, median 40 years. Periods of less than 25 years are very rare. In our series we found 5 cases with 5, 8, 10, 19, 20 years. Short latency periods were usually found in those people who left their wood-working jobs and continued working elsewhere. Persons who worked exclusively as woodworkers had markedly longer latency periods.

If there was an additional exposure to wood preservatives, solvents, lacquers or dust of plywood and chipboards we noticed shorter latency periods too. One group of woodworkers was completely missed in our series: those persons who definitely had been exposed to dust of untreated hard woods like builders of frames or wooden toys. In those patients who worked with preservatives and plywood or chipboard we found more tumours of high grade malignancy than in the others. Thus we cannot exclude the possibility that there are other substances in addition to wood dust which work as promoting factors.

Clinical Behaviour

Nasal adenocarcinomas are characterized by an indolent progression with early symptoms mimicking nonspecific nasal disease (table 4). 72% of the patients suffered from nasal obstruction several months before diagnosis. 27% had rhinorrhoea. Nose bleed was found in more than 40%. Only 15% noticed the more severe eye symptoms like double vision, exophthalmos or loss of vision. Most patients came to the clinic with an advanced

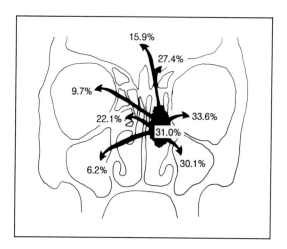

Fig. 2. Tumour expansion at diagnosis of 123 cases of nasal adenocarcinoma after wood dust exposure.

Table 4. Symptoms of 123 persons with nasal adenocarcinoma after wood dust exposure

Symptom	Frequency, %	Duration before diagnosis	
		median	range
Nasal obstruction	72.4	5 m	1 m–7 y
Epistaxis	40.7	5 m	2 w–3 y
Rhinorrhoea	27.6	4 m	2 w–5 y
Sinusitis	15.4	6 m	1 m–7 y
Headache	18.7	4 m	1 m–2 y
Eye symptoms	15.4	2 m	1 w–6 m
Smell disorder	3.3	6 m	2 m–4 y

stage of the disease because neither they themselves nor their physicians had thought of a tumour.

Figure 2 shows the extension of the tumours at the time of diagnosis. The adenocarcinomas originated exclusively in the region of the middle turbinate and the adjacent ethmoidal region. Only 31% of the tumours had been restricted to this area at the time of diagnosis. In more than one third of the cases the tumour was found in the ipsilateral orbit. 27% of the

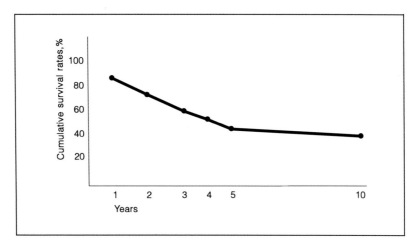

Fig. 3. Cumulative survival rates of 123 cases of nasal adenocarcinoma after wood dust exposure.

tumours reached the frontal base of the skull and in 15% there was even an intracerebral growth. Bilateral expansion was seen in 22%.

Lymph node metastases were found only in advanced stages in 3 of 123 cases, 2 of them had in addition haematogenic metastases. The cumulative survival rate is declining continuously from 89% after 1 year to 62% after 3 years and 47% after 5 years (fig. 3). The survival rates of smokers and nonsmokers are markedly different. Whereas the 5-year survival rate of smokers is 41%, nonsmokers have a rate of 57%. Perhaps tobacco smoking is another promoting factor in interaction with wood dust.

Since these tumours are relatively slow growing but locally destructive the only promising therapy is an early surgical intervention with lateral rhinotomy and block resection of the tumour. Irradiation and chemotherapy do not seem to have any effect on the growth of nasal adenocarcinomas.

Prevention

Concerning tumour prevention we have to consider two aspects: the technical and the medical one. From the fact that we did not find one single case in our series who worked under conditions of low wood dust concentration, it must be inferred that we have to reduce wood dust emissions as far as possible. In Germany the threshold value for new licensed woodworking machines is 2 mg/m³. The medical part of prevention is much more difficult because we do not know either risk factors or precancerous lesions. In our series we did not find any correlation with preceding allergic, traumatic or inflammatory nasal disease.

Boysen [11] and Wilhelmsson et al. [12] supposed cuboidal metaplasia to be the actual precursor of adenocarcinoma. In our opinion it would be astonishing if a cylindrical cell adenocarcinoma developed from cylindrical cells via cuboidal metaplasia finally again to high cylindrical tumour cells. In 1 of our cases we found in the surrounding area of a microinvasive tumour a peripheral zone of adenocarcinoma in situ which followed the superficial structures and extended partially also into the excretory ducts of the nasal glands. These malignant cylindrical cells seemed to arise directly from the ciliated cylindrical cells without intermediate stage of cuboidal metaplasia [13]. Instead of preventive examinations we have to take care of an early diagnosis which is only possible if all persons at risk are examined periodically by nasal endoscopy.

In summary, this series of 123 woodworkers with nasal adenocarcinoma demonstrates that after exposure to oak and beech wood dust only a specific type of tumour arises resembling gastrointestinal adenocarcinomas. These tumours originate from the nasal mucosa only in a circumscript region surrounding the middle turbinate. Detailed features of the carcinogenicity are not clear. Further experimental studies are being performed to find out which substances act as carcinogenic agents or promoting factors.

References

1   Hill JP: Cautions against the Immoderate Use of Snuff. London, Baldwin & Jackson, 1761.
2   Personal information from the German Industrial Injuries Insurance Institute.
3   Macbeth R: Malignant disease of the paranasal sinuses. J Laryngol Otol 1965;79: 592–612.
4   Mohtashamipur E, Norpoth K, Lühmann F: Cancer epidemiology of woodworking. J Cancer Res Clin Oncol 1989;115:503–515.
5   Schroeder HG: Adenokarzinome der inneren Nase und Holzstaubexposition. Sankt Augustin, Hauptverband der gewerblichen Berufsgenossenschaft e.V., 1989.
6   Wolf J: Untersuchung über bösartige Tumoren der Nase und ihre Beziehung zur Holzstaubexposition in der Bundesrepublik Deutschland. Sicherheitswissenschaftliche Monographien. Wuppertal, Gesellschaft für Sicherheitswissenschaften, 1988, vol 13.

7   Kleinsasser O, Schroeder HG: Adenocarcinomas of the inner nose after exposure to wood dust. Morphological findings and relationships between histopathology and clinical behavior in 79 cases. Arch Otorhinolaryngol 1988;245:1–15.

8   Kleinsasser O: Klassifikation und Verhalten der Adenokarzinome der Nase; in Majer EH, Zrunek M (eds): Aktuelles in der Otorhinolaryngologie, 1984. Stuttgart, Thieme, 1985, pp 88–89.

9   Kleinsasser O: Terminal tubulus adenocarcinoma of the nasal seromucous glands. A specific entity. Arch Otorhinolaryngol 1985;241:183–193.

10 Hadfield EH: A study of adenocarcinoma of the paranasal sinuses in woodworkers in the furniture industry. Ann R Coll Surg Engl 1970;46:301–319.

11 Boysen M: Histopathology of the nasal mucosa in furniture workers. Rhinology 1985;23:109–113.

12 Wilhelmsson B, Hellquist H, Olofsson J, et al: Nasal cuboidal metaplasia with dysplasia. Acta Otolaryngol (Stockh) 1985;99:641–648.

13 Kleinsasser O, Schroeder HG, Mayer-Brix J: Precancerous lesions in adenocarcinoma of the nose after exposure to wood dust. Arch Otorhinolaryngol; in press.

Priv.-Doz. Dr. H.-G. Schroeder, Universitäts-HNO-Klinik, Deutschhausstrasse 3, D-W-3550 Marburg (FRG)

Pfaltz CR, Arnold W, Kleinsasser O (eds): Bearing of Basic Research on Clinical Otolaryngology. Adv Otorhinolaryngol. Basel, Karger, 1991, vol 46, pp 116–123

Viruses in Cancers of the Head and Neck

Ethel-Michele de Villiers

Referenzzentrum für humanpathogene Papillomviren,
Deutsches Krebsforschungszentrum, Heidelberg, FRG

Viruses which have to date been associated with tumours of the head and neck are the Epstein-Barr virus (EBV) and human papillomaviruses (HPV).

The presence of the EBV DNA has been demonstrated in almost a 100% of samples of anaplastic nasopharyngeal carcinomas [1]. In vitro studies, to elucidate the exact mechanism by which the EBV may act in the process of malignant transformation in these tumours, have been hampered by the absence of a suitable cell culture system of these neoplasms.

The first HPV to be identified in a tumour of the mucosal tissue, i.e. in a condyloma acuminatum of the genital tract [2], was HPV 6. To date, 66 different types of HPVs have been identified and their DNA characterized. Of these, 30 HPV types have originally been isolated from mucosal tumours of either the genital tract or the head and neck region. The DNA of 2 out of the 30, HPV 13 [3] and HPV 32 [4], has subsequently been detected in the oral mucosa only. HPV 13 DNA has been found solely in lesions of focal epithelial hyperplasia, whereas HPV 32 DNA was isolated from such lesions, but also present in a case of oral papillomatosis [4]. HPV 11 originates from a laryngeal papilloma [5], HPV 30 from a laryngeal carcinoma [6] and HPV 57 from an inverted papilloma of the maxillary sinus [7]. The latter three HPVs were, upon further investigation, frequently found in tumours of the genital tract, i.e. in condylomata acuminata or in intraepithelial neoplasias.

Papillomaviruses in Anogenital Cancer

Zur Hausen [8] postulated that cervical cancer is related to a papillomavirus infection. Since then, the role of these viruses in the etiology of malignant, as well as benign tumours, has been examined in great detail, especially for HPVs associated predominantly with lesions of the genital tract. Although some of the types, e.g. HPV 6, 11, 42, 43, 44, 51 and 55, have been detected mainly in biopsies of condylomata acuminata or low degree intraepithelial neoplasias [9], they could be associated with certain carcinomas as well, as has been demonstrated for HPV 6 or HPV 11 in verrucous carcinomas and Buschke-Loewenstein tumours [10, 11]. HPV DNA is present in more than 90% of cases of high grade genital intraepithelial neoplasias and carcinomas, with HPV 16 being the most prevalent type found in carcinomas (50%), followed by HPV 18 (20%) and HPV 33 (10%) [12]. HPV 18 is very frequently found in adenocarcinomas of the cervix [13].

Genital HPV infections were widely spread and found in populations studied all over the world [12]. Examining cervical samples with normal cytology obtained from a population of women in Germany, 10–12% of the sexually active adults were positive for HPV DNA [14]. With repeated testing of the same individuals, the positivity increased to 35%.

HPV infection emerged as a necessary, but not sufficient factor for the malignant transformation [15]. Not only are these HPVs present in these tumours, but in vitro studies could demonstrate that certain sections or genes (E6 and E7 open reading frames) of the double-stranded DNA molecule could transform rodent cells [16–18] and immortalize human foreskin and cervical keratinocytes [19–21]. The growth of HPV 16 DNA transfected primary keratinocytes on the raft tissue culture system allowing the differentiation of these cells, leads to the induction of Bowenoid type changes [22]. By heterografting HPV 11 transfected human cervical cells under the renal capsule of nude mice, Kreider et al. [23] demonstrated in vivo the role of HPV 11 in the development of condyloma acuminatum.

The additional genetical events, which are necessary in the chain of reactions taking place in the development of anogenital carcinogenesis, are increasingly being understood [24]. A host cell-mediated intracellular control appears to down-regulate the transforming HPV genes (E6 and E7 ORF) in the normal replicating cell. In a malignantly transformed cell, this suppressing host control seems to be disrupted [25], leading to the expression and translation of the E6-E7 genes of the HPV present in the cell. In vitro data shows that the E7-E6 genes play a role in the proliferation of cervical carcinoma cells and in the maintenance of the malignant phenotype [26]. In vivo studies in immunoincompetent mice, point to the activation of the normal suppressing host control by humoral factors [27]. Similarly, these normal suppressing host control genes could be completely inactivated by mutagenic events of humoral cofactors, such as mutagenic metabolites of secondary bacterial infections, smoke and alcohol [24]. These latter are likely to determine the different geographic incidence rates of cervical cancer. As the development of the tumour is a monoclonal event, the relatively low number of HPV-infected individuals developing genital carcinomas could be explained by the extremely low risk of all the above-mentioned events taking place within one cell.

Papillomaviruses in Tumours of the Head and Neck

'... if cervical cancer were related to condyloma virus infection, consideration of cancer of the oral cavity, the lung, and the bladder should be included in such a discussion' [28].

As in the genital tract, HPV infection is very frequently associated with benign lesions of the oral cavity and upper respiratory tract [9]. HPV 11 was isolated from a laryngeal papilloma [5]. Various reports demonstrated the frequency of the presence of HPV 6 or HPV 11 DNA in such tumours. In recent reports [29–32], 75–100% of laryngeal papillomas contained either HPV 6 or HPV 11 DNA.

The majority of oral papillomatoses contain either HPV 6 or HPV 11 DNA [33], although the detection of the DNA of any of the known HPV types could thus far not be detected in papillomas of the palate [34; de Villiers and Hotz, unpubl. results]. As mentioned previously, an infection with HPV 13 or HPV 32 seems to develop differently. These two viruses have only been demonstrated in oral lesions, i.e. mainly in focal epithelial hyperplasias [3, 4, 35], with HPV 32 occasionally present in an oral papillomatosis.

From an inverted papilloma of the maxillary sinus, HPV 57 DNA could be isolated and characterized [7]. After sequencing the HPV 57 DNA genome, a 83% nucleotide homology to the HPV 2 DNA could be established [36]. Other investigators demonstrated HPV 6, 11 or HPV 16 in nasal inverted papillomas [29, 37–39].

Infection of the oral mucosa with HPV types frequently found in genital infections may not be uncommon, although these infections most probably remain subclinical [40]. Infection with any of the other HPVs could occur as well. Greenspan et al. [41] reported the presence of HPV 7 DNA in a large percentage of oral papillomatous lesions from patients infected with the human immunodeficiency virus (HIV). This HPV 7 has only very rarely been found in lesions other than verrucae vulgares on the hands of people handling meat [42, 43]. This infection of HPV 7 in the oral cavity, which was not geographically localized, underlines the notion that many of the HPV infections remain latent or subclinical. Only under certain circumstances, e.g. certain immunosuppressing events, does the virus become activated resulting in cell proliferation and virus production [44]. The increased incidence of tumours of the upper respiratory tract in renal transplant recipients point to a similar event [45].

The demonstration of HPV DNA in malignant tumours of the head and neck has been less successful. As previously reported [33], the application of different DNA detection techniques by the different investigators has led to contradictory results. Even more so with the advent of the highly sensitive polymerase chain reaction (PCR). Additional studies are required to clarify the discrepancy between results obtained using the PCR [46] and other methods [33].

The number of biopsies obtained from malignant lesions containing any of the known HPV types remain small. HPV 16 DNA is relatively often present in carcinomas, e.g. in a maxillary carcinoma, as well as in a tonsillar carcinoma [47], a laryngeal carcinoma [48] and carcinoma of the floor of the mouth and tongue carcinoma [49; de Villiers, unpubl. results]. These are, however, single cases of large numbers of biopsies tested and the majority of such lesions remain negative for the presence of any specific HPV type.

HPV-related DNA sequences have been detected in malignant tumours of varying origin [33, 50], although again, the percentage of lesions containing such DNA sequences remains low. In these cases, the DNA has to be isolated and characterized to determine wether these are specific HPV DNA sequences.

The detection of specific HPV DNA has been hampered by the absence of adequate DNA probes. The presence of koilocytosis is a specific histological criterium for an infection by any HPV. Kashima et al. [51] reported the presence of koilocytosis in 90% of carcinoma and 50% of leukoplakia specimens taken from the oral cavity. However, only 7 of 74 oral cavity squamous cell carcinomas and 1 of 45 leukoplakia specimens contained detectable HPV DNA. This suggests that, as histological evidence points to the presence of HPV DNA, the HPV types predominantly responsible for the development of such malignant lesions have not to date been identified. Although the mechanism of action of an HPV infection in the malignant transformation event is most probably the same in the mucosa of the oral cavity and upper respiratory tract as in the genital mucosa, such studies could only progress upon identification of these as yet unknown HPV types.

References

1 zur Hausen H: DNA viruses in human cancer: Biochemical approaches. Cancer Res 1976;36:414–416.
2 Gissmann L, zur Hausen H: Partial characterization of viral DNA from human genital warts (condylomata acuminata). Int J Cancer 1980;25:605–609.
3 Pfister H, Hettich I, Runne U, Gissmann L, Chilf GN: Characterization of human papillomavirus type 13 from lesions of focal epithelial hyperplasia. J Virol 1983;47:363–366.
4 Beaudenon S, Praetorius F, Kremsdorf D, Lutzner M, Worsae N, Petnau-Arnaudet G, Orth G: A new type of human oral papillomavirus associated with focal epithelial hyperplasia. J Invest Dermatol 1987;88:130–135.
5 Gissmann L, Diehl V, Schultz-Coulon H, zur Hausen H: Molecular cloning and characterization of human papillomavirus DNA from a laryngeal papilloma. J Virol 1982;44:393–400.
6 Kahn T, Schwarz E, zur Hausen H: Molecular cloning and characterization of the DNA of the new human papillomavirus (HPV 30) from a laryngeal carcinoma. Int J Cancer 1986;37:61–65.
7 de Villiers E-M, Hirsch-Behnam A, von Knebel Doeberitz C, Neumann C, zur Hausen H: Two newly identified human papillomavirus types (HPV 40 and 57) isolated from mucosal lesions. Virology 1989;171:248–253.
8 zur Hausen H: Condylomata acuminata and human genital cancer. Cancer Res 1976;36:530.
9 de Villiers E-M: Heterogeneity of the human papillomavirus group. J Virol 1989;63:4898–4903.
10 Boshart M, zur Hausen H: Human papillomaviruses (HPV) in Buschke-Loewenstein tumors: Physical state of the DNA and identification of a tandem duplication in the non-coding region of a HPV 6-subtype. J Virol 1986;58:963–966.
11 Randall RF, Sedlacek TV, Hunt J, Jenson AB, Kurman RJ, Lancaster WD: Verrucous carcinoma of the vulva associated with an unusual type 6 papillomavirus. Obstet Gynecol 1986;67i:70S–75S.
12 zur Hausen H: Papillomaviruses as carcinomaviruses; in Klein G (ed): Advances in Viral Oncology. New York, Raven Press, 1989, vol 8, pp 1–26.

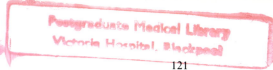

13   Tase T, Okagaki T, Clark BA, Manias DA, Ostrow RS, Twiggs LB, Faras AJ: Human papillomavirus types and localization in adenocarcinoma and adenosquamous carcinoma of the uterine cervix: A study by in situ hybridization. Cancer Res 1988;48: 993–998.

14   de Villiers E-M, Wagner D, Schneider A, Wesch H, Miklaw H, Wahrendorf J, Papendick U, zur Hausen H: Human papillomavirus infections in women with and without abnormal cervical cytology. Lancet 1987;ii:703–706.

15   zur Hausen H: Intracellular surveillance of persisting viral infections: Human genital cancer results from deficient cellular control of papillomavirus gene expression. Lancet 1986;ii:489–491.

16   Yasumoto S, Burkardt A, Doniger J, DiPaolo J: Human papillomavirus type 16 DNA-induced malignant transformation of NIH3T3 cells. J Virol 1986;57:572–577.

17   Bedell MA, Jones KH, Laimins LA: The E6-E7 region of human papillomavirus type 18 is sufficient for transformation of NIH3T3 and Rat-1 cells. J Virol 1987;61: 3635–3640.

18   Matlashewski G, Schneider J, Banks L, Jones N, Murray A, Crawford L: Human papillomavirus type 16 cooperates with activated ras in transforming primary cells. EMBO J 1987;6:1741–1746.

19   Dürst M, Dzarlieva-Petrusevska RT, Boukamp P, Fusenig NE, Gissmann L: Molecular and cytogenetic analysis of immortalized human primary keratinocytes obtained after transfection with human papillomavirus type 16 DNA. Oncogene 1987; 1:251–256.

20   Pirisi L, Yasumoto S, Feller M, Doniger J, DiPaolo J: Transformation of human fibroblasts and keratinocytes with human papillomavirus type 16 DNA. J Virol 1987;61:1061–1066.

21   Kaur P, McDougall JK: Characterization of primary human keratinocytes transformed by human papillomavirus type 18. J Virol 1988;62:1917–1924.

22   McCance DJ, Kopan R, Fuchs E, Laimins L: Human papillomavirus type 16 alters human epithelial cell differentiation in vitro. Proc Natl Acad Sci 1988;85:7169–7173.

23   Kreider J, Howett M, Wolfe SA, Bartlett G, Zaino R, Sedlacek T, Mortel R: Morphological transformation in vivo of human uterine cervix with papillomavirus from condylomata acuminata. Nature (Lond) 1985;317:639–641.

24   zur Hausen H: Papillomaviruses in anogenital cancer as a model to understand the role of viruses in human cancers. Cancer Res 1989;49:4677–4681.

25   Rösl F, Dürst M, zur Hausen H: Selective suppression of human papillomavirus transcription in non-tumorigenic cells by 5-azacytidine. EMBO J 1988;7:1321–1328.

26   von Knebel Doeberitz M, Oltersdorf T, Schwarz E, Gissmann L: Correlation to modified human papillomavirus early gene expression with altered growth properties in C4-1 cervical carcinoma cells. Cancer Res 1988;48:3780–3786.

27   Bosch FX, Schwarz E, Boukamp P, Fusenig NE, Bartsch D, zur Hausen H: Suppression in vivo of human papillomavirus type 18 E6-E7 gene expression in nontumorigenic HeLa × fibroblast hybrid cells. J Virol 1990;64:4743–4754.

28   zur Hausen H: Human papillomaviruses and their possible role in squamous cell carcinomas. Curr Top Microbiol 1977;78:1–30.

29 Furuta Y, Inuyama Y, Nagashima K: Detection of human papillomavirus genome in nasopharyngeal papillomas using digoxigenin labeled DNA probes. Nippon Jibiinkoka Gakkai Kaiho 1989;92:2055–2063.

30 Levi JE, Delcelo R, Alberti VN, Torloni H, Villa LL: Human papillomavirus DNA in respiratory papillomatosis detected by in situ hybridization and the polymerase chain reaction. Am J Pathol 1989;135:1179–1184.

31 Brandsma JL, Lewis AJ, Abramson A, Manos MM: Detection and typing of papillomavirus DNA in formaldehyde-fixed paraffin-embedded tissue. Arch Otolaryngol Head Neck Surg 1990;116:844–848.

32 Duggan MA, Lim M, Gill MJ, Inoue M: HPV DNA typing of adult-onset respiratory papillomatosis. Laryngoscope 1990;110:639–642.

33 de Villiers E-M: Papilloma virus in cancers and papillomas of the aerodigestive tract. Biomed Pharmacother 1989;43:31–36.

34 Seoane Leston JM, Sanchez Lopez M, Aguado Santos A, Garcia Varela L, Romero Mendez A, Esparza Gomez G: Detection of human papillomavirus antigens in papillomatous lesions of the palate. Av Odontoestomatol 1989;5:279–282.

35 Garlick JA, Calderon S, Buchner A, Mitrani-Rosenbaum S: Detection of human papillomavirus (HPV) DNA in focal epithelial hyperplasia. J Oral Pathol Med 1989; 18:172–177.

36 Hirsch-Behnam A, Delius H, de Villiers E-M: A comparative sequence analysis of two human papillomavirus (HPV) types 2a and 57 (in press).

37 Respler DS, Jahn A, Pater A, Pater MM: Isolation and characterization of papillomavirus DNA from nasal inverting (Schneiderian) papillomas. Ann Otol Rhinol Laryngol 1987;96:170–173.

38 Brandwein M, Steinberg B, Thung S, Biller H, Dilorenzo T, Galli R: Human papillomavirus 6/11 and 16/18 in Schneiderian inverted papillomas. In situ hybridization with human papillomavirus RNA probes. Cancer 1989;63:1708–1713.

39 Bryan RL, Bevan IS, Crocker J, Young LS: Detection of HPV 6 and 11 in tumours of the upper respiratory tract using the polymerase chain reaction. Clin Otolaryngol 1990;15:177–180.

40 Kellokoski J, Syrjaenen S, Syrjaenen K, Yliskoski M: Oral mucosa changes in women with genital HPV infection. J Oral Pathol Med 1990;19:142–148.

41 Greenspan D, de Villiers E-M, Greenspan JS, de Souza YG, zur Hausen H: Unusual HPV types in oral warts in association with HIV infection. J Oral Pathol 1988;17: 482–487.

42 Orth G, Jablonska S, Favre M, Croissant O, Obalek S, Jarzabek-Chorzelska M, Jibard N: Identification of papillomaviruses in butcher's warts. J Invest Dermatol 1981;76:97–102.

43 de Villiers E-M, Neumann C, Oltersdorf T, Fierlbeck G, zur Hausen H: Butcher's wart virus (HPV 7) infections in non-butchers. J Invest Dermatol 1986;87:236–238.

44 de Villiers E-M: Prevalence of HPV 7 papillomas in the oral mucosa and facial skin of patients with human immunodeficiency virus. Arch Dermatol 1989;125:1590.

45 Bradford CR, Hoffman HT, Wolf GT, Carey TE, Baker SR, McClatchey KD: Squamous carcinoma of the head and neck in organ transplant recipients: possible role of oncogenic viruses. Laryngoscope 1990;100:190–194.

46 Perez-Ayala M, Ruiz-Cabello F, Esteban F, Concha A, Redondo M, Oliva MR, Cabrera T, Garrido F: Presence of HPV 16 sequences in laryngeal carcinomas. Int J Cancer 1990;46:8–11.

47 Ishibashi T, Matsushima S, Tsunokawa Y, Asai M, Nomura Y, Sigumura T, Terada M: Human papillomavirus DNA in squamous cell carcinoma of the upper aerodigestive tract. Arch Otolaryngol Head Neck Surg 1990;116:294–298.

48 Scheurlen W, Stremlau A, Giessmann L, Höhn D, Zenner HP, zur Hausen: Rearranged HPV 16 mulecules in an anal and in a laryngeal carcinoma. Int J Cancer 1986;38:671–676.

49 de Villiers E-M, Weidauer H, Otto H, zur Hausen H: Papillomavirus DNA in human tongue carcinomas. Int J Cancer 1985;36:575–578.

50 Brandsma JL, Abramson AL: Association of papillomavirus with cancers of the head and neck. Arch Otolaryngol Head Neck Surg 1989;115:621–625.

51 Kashima HK, Kutcher M, Kessis T, Levin LS, de Villiers E-M, Shah K: Human papillomavirus in squamous cell carcinoma, leukoplakia, lichen planus, and clinically normal epithelium of the oral cavity. Ann Otol Rhinol Laryngol 1990;99:55–61.

Ethel-Michele de Villiers, Referenzzentrum für humanpathogene Papillomviren, Deutsches Krebsforschungszentrum, Im Neuenheimer Feld 506, D-W–6900 Heidelberg (FRG)

Pfaltz CR, Arnold W, Kleinsasser O (eds): Bearing of Basic Research on Clinical Otolaryngology. Adv Otorhinolaryngol. Basel, Karger, 1991, vol 46, pp 124–133

International Variation in the Incidence of Cancer of the Upper Digestive and Respiratory Tract

Ole Møller Jensen [1]

Danish Cancer Registry, Institute of Cancer Epidemiology,
Danish Cancer Society, Copenhagen, Denmark

The science of epidemiology studies the distribution of diseases in human populations and uses its observations to seek for determinants. Variations between population groups have been of major importance for the identification of risk factors for cancer development, not least in the head and neck region. With few exceptions, all risk factors for cancer development in humans have first been identified by epidemiology.

The examination of international differences in the incidence of cancer has played an important role in epidemiology. The incidence of cancer of most sites varies by at least a factor of 10 from one region of the world to the other [1]. Such observations of international differences have contributed to the conclusion that most cancers develop in response to some exogenous exposure. This conclusion has been elegantly corroborated by studies of migrants whose cancer risks approach that of their new country when they migrate from high to low risk regions of the world.

This paper gives an overview of the magnitude of the problem of cancers of the oral cavity, pharynx and larynx, both worldwide and in the European Economic Community (EC). This is followed by a review of the international variation in the incidence of these tumours. The examination of such variations in the world rests on information compiled by the Inter-

[1] The assistance of Ms. Tenna Lytsen and Ms. Majken Bagger-Nielsen with preparation of the manuscript and graphics is gratefully acknowledged.

national Agency for Research on Cancer in collaboration with the International Association of Cancer Registries [1]. The description of the variations in the EC is based on recent estimates undertaken within the framework of The European Network of Cancer Registries, which operates under the auspices of the 'Europe against Cancer' programme of the EC [2].

Magnitude of the Problem

Parkin et al. [3] have estimated that there are about 6.4 million new cancer cases in the world each year. Out of these, some 361,000 new cases in men and 137,000 in women occur in the buccal cavity, pharynx, and larynx – this including cancer of the lips and salivary glands. These head and neck cancers account for 11% of all malignant diseases worldwide in men and about 4.4% in women.

The high proportion may come as a surprise to those with experience from the economically developed part of the world only. When Parkin et al. [3] looked at the distribution of cancer by site in the developed and the developing part of the world respectively, it became apparent that cancers of the oral cavity and pharynx rank among the leading cancers in the developing countries and much lower in developed regions. This is clearly reflected by the recent estimates of the cancer incidence which we have undertaken for the EC [4]. Cancer of the oral cavity, pharynx, and larynx constitutes some 40,000 new cases per year (35,800 men, 3,800 women) (table 1), corresponding to 5.5 and 0.7% of cancers of all sites in men and women, respectively.

Table 1. Tobacco- and alcohol-related upper digestive and respiratory tract cancers in the EC, 1980

ICD-9	Site	Males		Females	
		n	%	n	%
141, 143–145	mouth, tongue	5,900	0.9	1,600	0.3
146–149	pharynx	5,300	0.4	1,000	0.2
161	larynx	24,600	3.8	1,200	0.2
Total		35,800	5.5	3,800	0.7

Table 2. Worldwide difference in the incidence per 100,000[1] of cancer of the upper aerodigestive tract

ICD-9	Site	Highest		Lowest		Ratio
Males						
140	lip	15.1	Canada, New Foundland	0.1	Japan, Osaka	151.0
141	tongue	8.9	Martinique	0.4	China, Tianjin	22.3
142	salivary gland	3.0	Pacific Polynesian Isl.	0.4	USA, LA, Lat.	7.5
143–145	mouth	13.5	France, Bas-Rhin	0.5	Japan, Miyagi	27.0
146, 148–149	pharynx	31.3	France, Calvados	0.5	Iceland	62.6
147	nasopharynx	30.0	Hong Kong	0.3	UK, South West	100.0
160	nose, sinuses	2.2	Hungary, Vas	0.4	Spain, Zaragoza	5.5
161	larynx	17.8	Brazil, Sao Paolo	2.2	Japan, Miyagi	8.1
Females						
140	lip	1.6	Australia, Southern	0.1	UK, England & Wales	16.0
141	tongue	3.4	India, Bombay	0.2	Czechoslovakia, Slo.	17.0
142	salivary gland	2.0	UK, SE Scotland	0.2	UK, Birmingham	10.0
143–145	mouth	15.7	India, Bangalore	0.2	Japan, Miyagi	78.5
146, 148–149	pharynx	4.3	India, Bombay	0.2	Norway	21.5
147	nasopharynx	12.9	Hong Kong	0.1	USA, Iowa	129.0
160	nose, sinuses	1.8	Japan, Nagasaki	0.2	Canada, Brit. col.	9.0
161	larynx	2.7	USA, Connecticut, Blacks	0.2	Japan, Miyagi	13.5

[1] Rates based on 10 or more cases.

Cancer of the Buccal Cavity

Cancer of the buccal cavity comprises malignant neoplasms of the lip, tongue, and mouth which in the 9th Revision of the International Classification of Diseases [5] are numbered 140, 141, 143–145, respectively. In men there is a 20- to 30-fold variation in risk of these cancers around the world (table 2); for cancer of the lip it is more than 100-fold. The variation is in general less pronounced in women. From figure 1 it is apparent that the incidence of these tumours is particularly high in France and India. The high rates in India are seen for both men and women. This contrasts to the pattern elsewhere, where the male rates are some 2–4 times higher than in women.

Within the EC it has been estimated that there are 32,322 new cases of cancer (27,328 men, 4,994 women) of the buccal cavity and pharynx each year. The risk is much higher among the populations of Latin-speaking countries than in the populations of northern Europe (fig. 2). The interna-

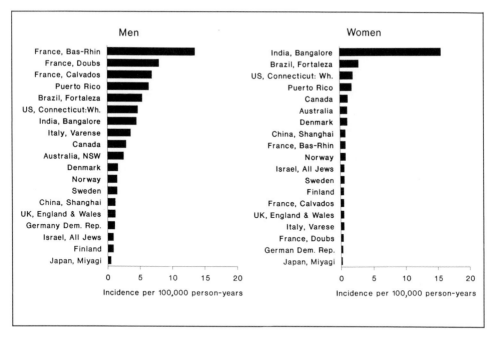

Fig. 1. International variation in the incidence of cancer of the oral cavity (ICD-9: 143–145).

tional differences for these diseases reflect the variation in smoking and alcohol consumption, which are the best documented determinants of cancers at these sites together with betel quid chewing in the Indian subcontinent [6–8]. To which extent dietary habits play an additional role needs clarification.

Cancer of the Pharynx

Cancer of the pharynx comprises tumours of the mesopharynx (ICD-9: 146), hypopharynx (ICD-9: 148), and pharynx unspecified (ICD-9: 149). To this adds cancer of the nasopharynx (ICD-9: 147), which biologically and functionally should rather be classified together with cancer of the nasal cavities and sinuses (see below).

Table 2 shows that there is a 60-fold difference between the male populations with the highest and lowest incidences on record in the world.

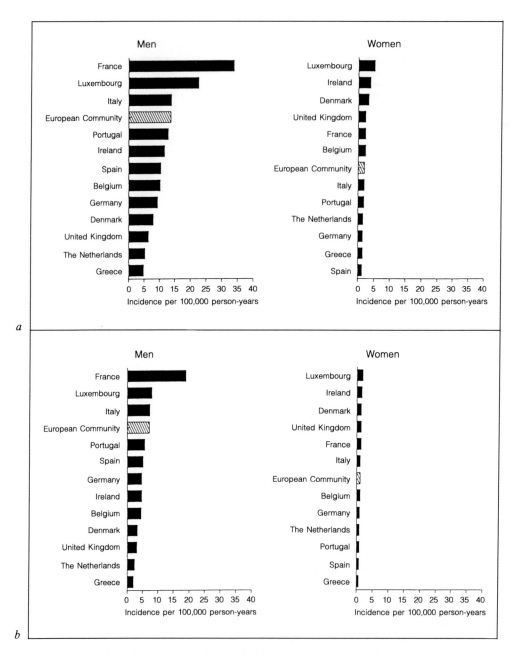

Fig. 2. Variation in the estimated incidence *a* and morality *b* of cancer of the buccal cavity and pharynx (ICD-9: 140–149) in the EC.

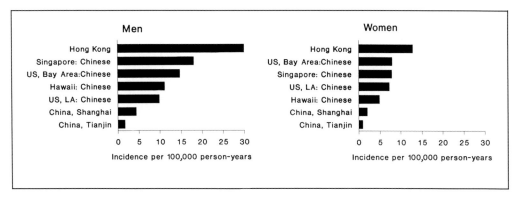

Fig. 3. International variation in the incidence of nasopharynx cancer (ICD-9: 147) among Chinese.

Among women the differences are less pronounced. In the EC there are an estimated 6,295 new cases each year with a 7 times higher risk of this disease in men than in women. The highest incidence rates are again seen in southern Europe for men, but northern European women have higher rates than women in the south. Among men in the Nordic countries, no geographical variation is seen apart from higher risks in the metropolitan areas [9]. The international variation as well as these urban-rural differences are in line with differences in alcohol and tobacco consumption. By contrast, the incidence among women in the Nordic countries is highest in the northern parts of Sweden where upper oesophageal cancer and hypopharyngeal cancer in the 1950s were associated with the Plummer-Vinson syndrome due to iron and riboflavin deficiency [10].

Cancer of the Nasopharynx, Nasal Cavities and Sinuses

Cancers of these sites are infrequent in most populations. The high incidence of nasopharynx cancer (ICD-9: 147) among Chinese has therefore been of particular interest for decades. Table 2 shows that the incidence among Chinese is 100 times higher than in the south west of the United Kingdom. The incidence is particularly high in southern China (Cantonese) and among Cantonese migrants to Singapore [11]. The incidence is also high irrespective of whether the Chinese live in mainland China or have migrated to, for example, Singapore or California [1] (fig. 3).

Table 3. Nasopharyngeal cancer in Greenland Inuit [from 13]

Period	Males		Females	
	incidence per 100,000 (WSR)[1]	relative risk[2]	incidence per 100,000 (WSR)	relative risk[2]
1958–62	2.4	6.0	3.9	36.4
1963–67	3.0	10.4	1.2	8.6
1968–72	19.0	37.3	5.1	23.6
1973–77	12.6	34.3	8.9	47.6
1978–82	10.1	15.4	10.4	53.3
1983–85	20.4	36.0	10.2	36.8
Hong Kong	30.0	–	12.9	–

[1] World standardized rate.
[2] Reference data: Denmark.

While this may indicate that host factors play an important aetiological role, exogenous factors have also been identified. The consumption of salted fish in early life seems to be an important risk factor for the development of this rare cancer [12]. In view of this, the observation of an equally high incidence of nasopharynx cancer among Inuit in Greenland [13] (table 3) as well as Alaska and Canada [14–16] is of interest. These areas may provide a setting for aetiological studies in a different ethnic group and in a different environment from southern China.

Cancers of the nasal cavities and sinuses (ICD-9: 160) are extremely rare in most populations (table 2).

Cancer of the Larynx

Cancer of the larynx (ICD-9: 161) comprises in the international classification of diseases the supraglottic, glottic, and subglottic parts. The delineation against the hypopharynx may be difficult, and may therefore hamper international comparisons. Table 2 shows a 35-fold variation between the highest and lowest incidence rates on record for men in the world. The highest rates are seen in various parts of France and among Blacks in the United States (fig. 4). Comparisons within the EC corrobo-

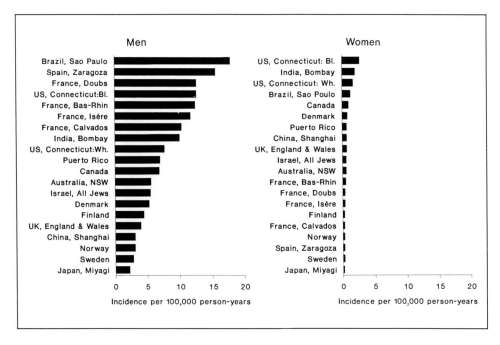

Fig. 4. International variation in the incidence of cancer of the larynx (ICD-9: 161).

rates the international variation in incidence with the highest rates in men in France, Italy, Spain, and Portugal and much lower rates in northern Europe. Among women the pattern is similar to that seen for cancer of the buccal cavity and pharynx with the highest rates in northern Europe. The international variation in incidence in men is in line with alcohol and tobacco being the major determinants of the disease in this sex [6, 7]; the pattern in women indicates that smoking habits are the major determinant of the presently observed pattern in that sex. To what extent dietary factors modify the distribution of laryngeal cancer is not known at present.

Conclusion

Cancer of the buccal cavity, pharynx, and larynx constitutes some 11% of all cancers in men and 4.4% in women in the world. There are large international differences, however, both in the importance of these cancers and in their relative frequencies within the upper aerodigestive tract region. On the international scale this is seen as large variations from one part of the world to the other. Such variations clearly point to exogenous factors as important causes.

There are clear similarities in the distribution of cancers of the mouth, tongue, pharynx and larynx, and in view of their neighbouring localizations it is not surprising that they share risk factors. The most important recognized causes of these cancers are tobacco and alcohol [6, 7], which have independent effects on the mucosa of these sites as well as a synergistic effect [6]. The international geographical patterns to a large degree reflect differences in alcohol and tobacco consumption. However, the oral cancer rate in India – high in both men and women – is a good example of the usefulness of the descriptive epidemiology for the identification of exceptions, which may provide clues to additional risk factors. In the case of oral cancer, betel quid chewing with tobacco has been isolated as the cause [8]. The geographical pattern of pharyngeal cancer among women in the Nordic countries is another exception which may warrant clarification by further studies of the role of diet in the origin of cancer of these sites.

International comparisons of cancer incidence have for decades pointed to the very high risk of nasopharyngeal cancer in Chinese and to studies of the causes of this cancer in this high risk population. The identification of a high incidence also in Inuit in the circumpolar area makes it possible to investigate the generalizability to other high risk populations of the Chinese results.

International descriptive studies of cancer of the upper aerodigestive tract have thus been of importance in pointing to factors, which in subsequent epidemiological investigations have been identified as causing cancer in this part of the body. Although the mechanism is not known by which tobacco and alcohol increases the risk of cancer development, there is today sufficient evidence that the elimination or diminution of these exposures will be followed by a decrease in the incidence of cancer.

References

1   Muir C, Waterhouse J, Mack T, Powell J, Whelan S (eds): Cancer Incidence in Five Continents, vol V: IARC Sci Publ No 88. Lyon, International Agency for Research on Cancer, 1987.
2   Commission of the European Community: Europe Against Cancer Action Plan, 1987–1989. Official Journal of the European Community. 1987;C50/01:1–58.

3   Parkin DM, Stjernswärd J, Muir CS: Cancer control. Estimates of the worldwide frequency of twelve major cancers. Bull World Health Org 1984;62:163–182.
4   Jensen OM, Estève J, Møller H, Renard H: Cancer in the European Community and its member states. EJC, in press.
5   World Health Organization: Manual of the International Statistical Classification of Diseases, Injuries, and Causes of Death. Geneva, WHO, 1977.
6   International Agency for Research on Cancer: IARC Monographs of the Evaluation of the Carcinogenic Risk of Chemicals to Humans, vol 38: Tobacco Smoking. Lyon, International Agency for Research on Cancer, 1986.
7   International Agency for Research on Cancer: IARC Monographs on the Evaluation of Carcinogenic Risks to Humans, vol 44: Alcohol Drinking. Lyon, International Agency for Research on cancer, 1988.
8   International Agency for Research on Cancer: IARC Monographs on the Evaluation of the Carcinogenic Risk of Chemicals to Humans, vol 37: Tobacco Habits Other than Smoking; Betel-Quid and Areca-Nut Chewing; and Some Related Nitrosamines. Lyon, International Agency for Research on Cancer, 1985.
9   Jensen OM, Carstensen B, Glattre E, Malker B, Pukkala E, Tulinius H: Atlas of Cancer Incidence in the Nordic Countries. Copenhagen, Nordic Cancer Union, 1988.
10 Wynder EL, Hultberg S, Jacobsson F, Bross IJ: Environmental factors in cancer of the upper alimentary tract. A Swedish study with special reference to Plummer-Vinson (Paterson-Kelly) syndrome. Cancer 1957;10:470–487.
11 Lee HP, Day NE, Shanmugaratnam K: Trends in Cancer Incidence in Singapore 1968–1982. IARC Sci Publ No 91. Lyon, International Agency for Research on Cancer, 1988.
12 Yu MC, Ho JH, Lai SH, Henderson BE: Cantonese-style salted fish as a cause of nasopharyngeal carcinoma: Report of a case-control study in Hong Kong. Cancer Res 1986;46:956–961.
13 Prener A, Nielsen NH, Storm HH, Hart Hansen JP, Jensen OM: Cancer in Greenland 1953–1985. APMIS, suppl, in press.
14 Nielsen NH, Mikkelsen F, Hart Hansen JP: Nasopharyngeal cancer in Greenland. Acta Pathol Microbiol Scand Sect A. 1977;85:850–858.
15 Lanier AP, Bender TR, Blot WJ, et al: Cancer incidence in Alaska natives. Int J Cancer 1976;18:409–412.
16 Schaefer O, Hildes JA, Medd LM, Cameron DG: The changing pattern of neoplastic disease in Canadian Eskimos. Can Med Assoc J 1975;112:1399–1404.

O.M. Jensen, MD, Danish Cancer Registry, Institute of Cancer Epidemiology, Danish Cancer Society, Rosenvængets Hovedvej 35, PO Box 639, DK-2100 Copenhagen (Denmark)

Pfaltz CR, Arnold W, Kleinsasser O (eds): Bearing of Basic Research on Clinical
Otolaryngology. Adv Otorhinolaryngol. Basel, Karger, 1991, vol 46, pp 134–144

Epidemiology of Head and Neck Cancer in Eastern Austria

H. Swoboda[1]

1st ENT Department (Head: Prof. Dr. *K. Ehrenberger*),
Vienna University, Vienna, Austria

Population-based investigations of cancer occurrence utilize centrally
collected medical and demographic data. In Austria, uniform data on population and death certificates are available from 1960 onwards at the Austrian Central Statistical Office. Nationwide registration of new cases was
initiated 1969 by the Austrian Cancer Registry. Obligation to report sub-
sists since 1970 [3] resulting in a satisfactory coverage of cases by the
beginning of the eighties. Population census, essential for detailed regional
differentiation, have been effectuated at 10-year intervals, the last in 1981.
In this paper, regional patterns of incidence of head and neck cancer from
1981 to 1985 in Eastern Austria and changes of mortality over the last
three decades are discussed, partly in comparison with lung cancer occurrence [7, 21–24].

Demographic Data

The term Eastern Austria denominates a coherent region numbering
3.2 million inhabitants enclosing Vienna, Lower Austria and Burgenland.
The region comprises the largest urban agglomeration and some of the
most pronouncedly agrarian regions of Austria. Following the 1981 Austrian census, 2.4 million inhabitants were allocated to urban communities

---

[1] For the layout of the graphs I am indebted to Mag. H. Plha, Austrian Central
Statistical Office.

exceeding 2,000 inhabitants and 0.8 to rural communities numbering up to 2,000 inhabitants, which results in an urban/rural population ratio of 3:1.

Incidence

Incidence values were computed as crude rates, i.e. new cases per 100,000 individuals per year, age-standardized and truncated standardized rates restricted to the age range 35–64 years, utilizing the standard population 'world' [28]. Sex ratios were calculated from crude rates, ratios of buccopharyngeal by lung cancer from age-standardized rates. Buccopharynx, i.e. oral cavity and oropharynx, on one side (ICD-9 141, 143–146, 149), and larynx and hypopharynx (ICD 161, 148) on the other were joined to two major ENT areas. This was done to compensate possible inaccuracies of the reported diagnoses. The other sites studied are lips (ICD 140), salivary glands (ICD 142), nasopharynx (ICD 147) and nasal and paranasal cavities and middle ears (ICD 160).

Results

In the quinquennium 1981–1985, cancer of the ENT section of the aerodigestive tract (ICD-9 140–149, 160, 161) accounted for 3.8% of all registered new cases, 6.3% in males and 1.3% in females. Age-standardized incidence rates of buccopharyngeal tumours amount to 7.1 male cases per 100,000 standard world population and 1.1 female cases. Larynx and hypopharynx exhibit cancer rates of 7.1 in males and 0.6 in females (table 1).

Incidence patterns of the two major ENT areas differed considerably by sex (table 1). Sex ratios were high, notably in cancer of larynx/hypopharynx. Regional distribution was opposite by sex, and more pronounced in women. In males it showed a rural accentuation of buccopharyngeal and an even repartition of laryngo-hypopharyngeal tumours. In females on the contrary there was a marked urban-rural gradient in buccopharyngeal as well as in laryngo-hypopharyngeal tumours.

Lung cancer presented in both sexes an urban predominance. In males it was small, and in females less pronounced than in the head and neck sites. Ratios of buccopharyngeal by lung tumours emphasize the rural accentuation of the former in males and inversely its urban predominance in females (table 2). Unlike these major so-called tobacco-related ENT

Table 1. Incidence and urban/rural ratios of cancer of oral cavity and oropharynx (ICD 141, 143–146, 149), larynx and hypopharynx (ICD 161, 148), lips (ICD 140), nasal and paranasal cavities and middle ears (ICD 160), nasopharynx (ICD 147), major salivary glands (ICD 142) and trachea, bronchi and lungs (ICD 162), by sex, Eastern Austria 1981–1985

Site	Sex	n	New cases per 100,000 and year			Urban/ rural ratio (world)	Sex ratio m/f (crude)
			world[1]	truncated[2]	crude		
Oral cavity/	m	685	7.1	18.7	9.2	0.8	4.4
oropharynx	f	181	1.1	2.3	2.1	2.4	
Larynx/	m	732	7.1	16.3	9.8	1	9.5
hypopharynx	f	88	0.6	1.1	1	3.5	
Lips	m	75	0.6	1	1	0.4	4.3
	f	20	0.06	0.03[3]	0.2	1	
Nasal and	m	34	0.3	0.6	0.5	1.1	0.9
paranasal cavities,	f	39	0.3	0.6	0.5	1.3	
middle ears							
Nasopharynx	m	54	0.6	1.4	0.7	0.9	1.8
	f	34	0.3	0.5	0.4	0.9	
Major salivary	m	68	0.6	0.9	0.9	0.8	1.2
glands	f	63	0.4	0.5	0.7	1.2	
Trachea, bronchi	m	4,968	42.4	68.5	66.7	1.2	3.7
and lungs	f	1,569	8.1	13.6	18.3	1.9	

[1] World = age-standardized rates 'world'.
[2] Truncated = age-standardized rates of the age group 35–64 years.
[3] n < 10.

Table 2. Ratios of buccopharyngeal (B) by lung tumour incidence (L), from age-standardized rates, by sex, Eastern Austria 1981–1985

B/L	Urban	Rural
Males	0.15	0.22
Females	0.14	0.11

areas, nasal, paranasal and tubotympanic cavities, nasopharynx and salivary glands exhibit low incidence values, even regional distribution and low male preponderance (table 1).

Mortality

Whereas incidence computation was suitable for cross-sectional study of regional distribution, longitudinal analysis of temporal developments had to recur to mortality data. Comparison of our hospital data with regional mortality substantiated a good accordance of long-term age-specific time trends [22, 23]. The grouping of the two main head and neck areas for mortality statistics into lip, mouth and pharynx (ICD 140–149) and larynx (ICD 160) slightly differs from that for incidence study. Mortality data were computed as annual age-standardized rates using the standard 'world', age-specific rates and cohort analysis [4, 28]. This later consists in a diagonal rearrangement of quinary-quinquennial age-specific rates relating selectively to birth cohorts of individuals born in successive periods designated by their central year of birth. Many of the resultant age curves remain fragmentary correspondingly to the limits of the period observed [4].

Results

The most conspicuous feature of mortality is the steady increase of male mouth and pharynx cancer rates from the sixties onwards. Lung cancer in males by contrast has been declining from the mid-seventies onwards (fig. 1). In females a recent increase in mouth and pharynx cancer follows with latency a steady increase of lung cancer (fig. 2). Larynx cancer mortality developments are less distinct (fig. 1, 2). Age-specific curves in males suggest a double wave-shaped cohort effect. Increasing rates in old age groups are followed by diminishing rates in middle age groups, notably in lung cancer, and in young age groups a rise is seen again, especially in mouth and pharynx malignancies (fig. 3, 4). This generation effect is best documented by cohort analysis: early cohorts born up to 1900, traceable only in advanced age, show successively increasing rates. Cohorts born around 1905–1915 show decreasing rates, which in lung cancer accounts for the decrease of mortality. Cohorts born after 1915–1920 exhibit increasing rates of mouth and pharynx cancer. A similar increase in lung cancer is much later and smaller (fig. 5, 6).

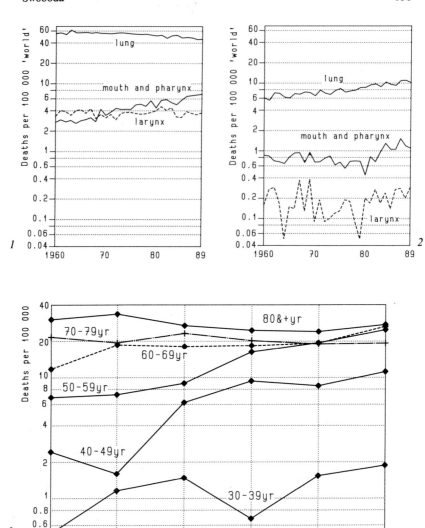

Fig. 1. Mortality from cancer of mouth and pharynx, larynx and lung, annual age-standardized rates, males, Eastern Austria 1960–1989.

Fig. 2. Mortality from cancer of mouth and pharynx, larynx and lung, annual age-standardized rates, females, Eastern Austria 1960–1989.

Fig. 3. Cancer of mouth and pharynx, age-specific mortality, 10-year age groups, males, Eastern Austria 1960–1989.

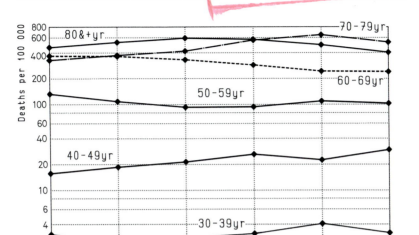

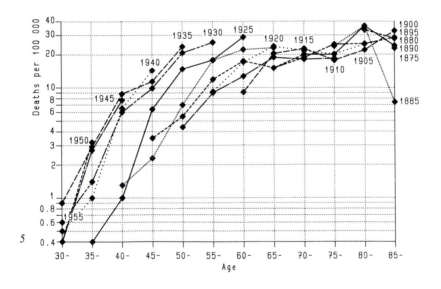

Fig. 4. Lung cancer, age-specific mortality, 10-year age groups, males, Eastern Austria 1960–1989.

Fig. 5. Cancer of mouth and pharynx, mortality, cohort analysis, males, Eastern Austria 1960–1989. Designation by central year of birth.

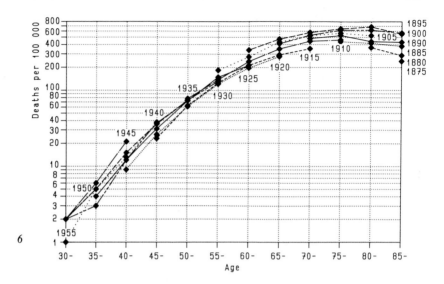

6

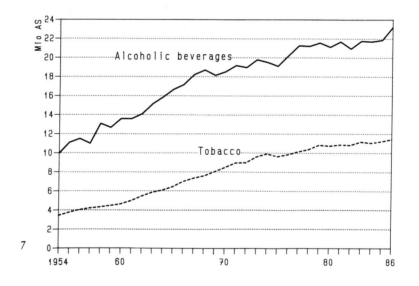

7

Fig. 6. Lung cancer, mortality, cohort analysis, males, Eastern Austria 1960–1989. Designation by central year of birth.

    Fig. 7. Expenditures of private households (natives), Austria 1954–1986, in million Austrian Shillings at 1976 prices [Mag. R. Schwarzl, Austrian Central Statistical Office].

Discussion

Hospital data compiled in 1880 by Gurlt [11] from Vienna demonstrate that head and neck and lung cancer were rare at that time. The 1981–1985 Eastern Austria incidence figures compare fairly well with those given by other Central European registries. They are higher than many Northern European rates and substantially lower than the respective rates reported by Southwestern European countries of Latin origin [12, 26, 28]. In the head-neck portion of the aerodigestive tract (ICD 140–149, 160, 161), 86 % of malignant neoplasms in men and 63 % in women affected oral cavity, oro-, hypopharynx or larynx (ICD 141, 143–146, 148, 149, 161) [21, 24]. Extant studies of mortality time trends in Austria unfortunately do not contain data pertaining to head and neck sites [1, 6]. Unpublished data from a recent survey upon causes of death evidenced in males a rise of mortality from mouth and pharynx cancer in Eastern Austria by 17 % within 10 years, but the recent increase of female rates did not yet appear [2]. Rising occurrence of buccopharyngeal cancer is a common observation in industrialized countries [12, 15, 18].

As concerns head and neck cancer, today's knowledge, elaborated on case-control level, imputes exogenous risk enhancement mainly to chronic tobacco and alcohol abuse, especially when combined [5, 13, 14, 16, 19, 20, 26, 27, 29–31]. Cross-correlations to socioeconomic and educational status, regional life-style customs and other parameters have been investigated [5, 7, 13, 20, 25, 30, 31]. European south-north gradients of head and neck cancer occurrence and of larynx/lung ratios have been related to respective customary alcohol consumption figures [26].

Synoptically the presented observations may point to a common denominator suggesting a growing influence of alcohol consumption upon tobacco-related cancer occurrence: (1) Buccopharyngeal tumour incidence in males coincides better with regional alcohol consumption patterns than with those of tobacco use. Whereas tobacco consumption is still higher in urban areas, alcohol consumption in males in Eastern Austria is higher in rural areas [8–10, 17]. (2) Within tobacco-related aerodigestive tract cancer the proportion of mouth and pharynx tumours has been growing steadily. (3) Our hospital data indicate increasing numbers of male hypopharyngeal carcinomas [22]. (4) A steady rise of expenditures for alcoholic beverages and tobacco since the fifties is paralleled in males rather by mouth and pharynx than by lung cancer time trends (fig. 7). (5) Regional distribution of mortality from the joined two main ENT areas (ICD 140–149, 161) correlated in both sexes with that of mortality from liver cirrhosis, but not with regional cigarette consumption patterns [7].

Alcohol should be accounted for as an indicator in epidemiology of tobacco-related cancer, and underlying sociocultural patterns and their relationship to risk-increasing habits should further be investigated.

Conclusion

(1) Incidence of head and neck and lung cancer between 1981 and 1985 in Eastern Austria exhibited sex-specific regional distribution patterns: (a) In males, rural incidence rates of lip cancer and of oral cavity and oropharynx tumours were higher than urban ones. Lung tumour incidence was slightly higher in urban than in rural areas. (b) In females, cancer incidence of oral cavity and oropharynx, larynx and hypopharynx and lung showed a pronounced urban-rural gradient, steeper in head-neck than in lung tumours. (c) Cancer of lips, oral cavity, pharynx, larynx and lung showed in high male preponderance. (d) Incidence rates of cancer of nasal and paranasal cavities, middle ear, nasopharynx and salivary glands were low, with small urban-rural differences and little male preponderance.

(2) Long-term mortality from 1960 to 1989 presented in males a steady increase of mouth and pharynx cancer, no constant trend in larynx tumours and a decrease in lung cancer. A double wave-shaped cohort effect was best recognizable in mouth and pharynx and in lung tumours. Successively increasing rates of younger cohorts produced the increase of mortality from mouth and pharynx cancer. Decreasing rates in middle-aged cohorts caused the diminution of lung cancer mortality whereas increase in the young was late and small.

In females, mouth and pharynx cancer rose sharply by the beginning of the eighties, lung cancer had been rising steadily over the last three decades, and larynx cancer rates remained constantly low.

References

1   Austrian Central Statistical Office: Österreichischer Todesursachenatlas 1978/84. Wien, Österreichische Staatsdruckerei, 1989.
2   Austrian Central Statistical Office: unpubl. data.
3   Bundesgesetzblatt für die Republik Österreich 1969/138, 1969/425 und 1978/59.

4 Case RAM: Cohort analysis of mortality rates as an historical or narrative technique. Br J Prev Soc Med 1956;10:159–171.

5 Elwood JM, Pearson JCG, Skippen DH, Jackson SM: Alcohol, smoking, social and occupatinal factors in the aetiology of cancer of the oral cavity, pharynx and larynx. Int J Cancer 1984;34:603–612.

6 Friedl H-P: Trendanalyse der Sterblichkeit in Österreich in den Jahren 1969 bis 1984 nach Todesursachen. Statistische Nachrichten 1986;41:449–453.

7 Friedl H-P, Swoboda H: Sex-specific cancer incidence related to life-style risks in urban and rural areas of Austria. Poster, Annual IACR Meeting, Hamburg, Aug 13–15, 1990.

8 Friedl H-P: Rauchgewohnheiten und Bildungsniveau: Statistische Nachrichten 1987;42:460–463.

9 Friedl H-P: Rauchgewohnheiten und sozioökonomische Stellung. Statistische Nachrichten 1987;42:553–558.

10 Friedl H-P: Regionale Aspekte des Rauchens. Statistische Nachrichten 1987;42: 394–397.

11 Gurlt E: Beiträge zur chirurgischen Statistik. Arch Klin Chir 1880;25:421–469.

12 Hakulinen T, Andersen Aa, Malker B, Pukkala E, Schou G, Tulinius H: Trends in Cancer Incidence in the Nordic Countries. A Collaborative Study of the Five Nordic Cancer Registries. Helsinki, Nordic Cancer Registries, 1986.

13 Jensen OM: Cancer morbidity and causes of death among Danish brewery workers. Int J Cancer 1979;23:454–463.

14 Kissin B, Kaley MM, Su WH, Lerner R: Head and neck cancer in alcoholics. JAMA 1973;224:1174–1177.

15 Kurihara M, Aoki K, Tominaga S: Cancer Mortality Statistics in the World. Nagoya, University of Nagoya Press, 1984.

16 Luce D, Guenel P, Leclerc A, et al: Alcohol and tobacco consumption in cancer of the mouth, pharynx and larynx: a study of 316 female patients. Laryngoscope 1988; 98:313–316.

17 Mader R, Mittendorfer Ch, Pavlis L, Springer A: Österreichische Trinksitten. Konsumation – Einstellung – Gefährdung. Schriftenreihe des Ludwig-Boltzmann-Institutes für Suchtforschung. Wien, Brüder Hollinek, 1981, vol 4, p 39.

18 Neumann G: Bösartige Neubildungen von Lippe, Mundhöhle, Rachen, Nase, Ohr und Kehlkopf. Eine deskriptiv-epidemiologische Untersuchung. HNO 1988;36: 345–354.

19 Rothman KJ: The effect of alcohol consumption on risk of cancer of the head and neck. Laryngoscope 1978;88:51–55.

20 Schwartz D, Flamant R, Lellouch J, Denoix P: Results of a French survey on the role of tobacco, particularly inhalation, in different cancer sites. J Natl Cancer Inst 1961; 29:1085–1108.

21 Swoboda H, Friedl H-P: Incidence of cancer of the respiratory and upper digestive tract in urban and rural Eastern Austria; submitted for publication.

22 Swoboda H, Neumann H, Cartellieri M: Änderungen des Erkrankungsalters der Karzinome des Hypopharynx und des Larynx seit 1960. HNO 1989;37:85–91.

23 Swoboda H, Neumann H, Cartellieri M: Häufigkeit und Erkrankungsalter der Karzinome der Mundhöhle und des Mesopharynx. HNO 1989;37:338–342.

24   Swoboda H, Neumann H, Cartellieri M: Zur Epidemiologie bösartiger Neubil-
      dungen des Atmungs- und oberen Verdauungstraktes in Ostösterreich. Laryngol
      Rhinol Otol 1990;69:123–130.
25   Tuyns AJ, Audigier JC: Double wave cohort increase for oesophageal and laryngeal
      cancer in France in relation to reduced alcohol consumption during the Second
      World War. Digestion 1976;14:197–208.
26   Tuyns AJ, Estève J, Raymond L, et al: Cancer of the larynx/hypopharynx, tobacco
      and alcohol: IARC international case-control study. Int J Cancer 1988;41:483–
      491.
27   Vincent RG, Marchetta F: The relationship of the use of tobacco and alcohol to
      cancer of the oral cavity, pharynx or larynx. Am J Surg 1963;106:501–505.
28   Waterhouse J: Cancer Incidence in Five Continents. Lyon, IARC, 1982, vol 4, pp
      671 ff.
29   Wynder EL, Bross IJ: Aetiological factors in mouth cancer. Br Med J 1957;i:1137–
      1171.
30   Wynder EL, Stellman SD: Comparative epidemiology of tobacco-related cancers.
      Cancer Res 1977;37:4608–4622.
31   Wynder EL, Covey LS, Mabuchi K, Mushinski M: Environmental factors in cancer
      of the larynx. A second look. Cancer 1976;38:1591–1601.

Dr. Herwig Swoboda, 1. HNO-Klinik der Universität Wien, Lazarettgasse 14,
A–1090 Wien (Austria)

Pfaltz CR, Arnold W, Kleinsasser O (eds): Bearing of Basic Research on Clinical
Otolaryngology. Adv Otorhinolaryngol. Basel, Karger, 1991, vol 46, pp 145–156

Cancer of the Endolarynx, Epilarynx and Hypopharynx in South-Western Europe: Assessment of Tumoral Origin and Risk Factors

W. Lehmann[a], *L. Raymond*[b], *F. Faggiano*[b,c], *H. Sancho-Garnier*[d],
F. Blanchet[e], *A. Del Moral*[f], *L. Zubiri*[g], *B. Terracini*[c], *F. Berrino*[h],
G. Pequignot[i], *J. Esteve*[j], *A. Tuyns*[j]

[a] Clinic of Otolaryngology, Head and Neck Surgery, Cantonal University Hospital,
Geneva, Switzerland; [b] Geneva Tumor Registry and Preventive Medical
Department, Geneva, Switzerland; [c] Biomedical Science and Human Oncology
Department, Epidemiology of Tumors, University of Torino, Italy;
[d] Gustave-Roussy Institute, Villejuif, France; [e] François Baclesse Regional Center,
Caen, France; [f] Health Department, Pamplona, Spain; [g] Health Institute of the
Social Security, Zaragoza, Spain; [h] National Institute for Study and Treatment of
Tumors, Milan, Italy; [i] INSERM, Nutritive Section, Le Vésinet, France;
[j] International Agency for Research on Cancer, Lyon, France

The incidence of cancers of the larynx and hypopharynx varies considerably from one region of the world to the other. Regarding males, it is
particularly low in Scandinavia (< 1 case/year for 100,000 inhabitants).
The incidence rate is 4 in the UK, increasing to 8 in the USA, and seems to
be at least double, if not triple, in Latin America and South-Western
Europe [1]. Incidence is much lower in females than in males, with incidence rates varying between 1/7 and 1/30 [1]. The observed distribution of
alcohol consumption, which is with tobacco consumption the most important risk factor for these cancers, largely explains these geographic and sex
differences [2].

The variation in incidence of cancer at subsites of this anatomic
region is, however, difficult to explain. Existing descriptive data do not
allow these geographic differences to be interpreted with a sufficient degree
of accuracy. There are two reasons for this. On the one hand, the data by
country on risk factors, and especially on tobacco consumption, are not

detailed enough to allow confirmation of suggested hypotheses. On the other hand, the differences between countries are partly hidden by an inappropriate subdivision of the laryngopharyngeal region within the International Classification of Diseases [3] adopted by epidemiologists. According to this classification, epilarynx is classified partly with larynx, partly with hypopharynx and oropharynx. The identification of epilarynx is no better with the TNM classifications [4, 5] used by clinicians, since epilarynx is put together with supraglottic larynx. However, epilarynx corresponds to an anatomoclinical entity and a specific tumor site which makes its specification necessary [6–8]. Epidemiological studies based on individual consumption of alcohol and tobacco were carried out in North America [9, 10] where exposure to these risk factors differed widely, both in intensity and nature, from that observed in South-Western Europe. Therefore, a new ad hoc topographical classification was prepared for this case-control study. A detailed analysis of the risks associated with alcohol, tobacco, and diet have been published previously [11, 12].

The aim of the present study was to analyze the variations in the distribution of the site of tumoral origin and the specific role of alcohol and tobacco exposure regarding these variations, and the socioeconomic status.

Populations and Method

The study was carried out between 1979 and 1982, simultaneously in six regions covered by a cancer registry, i.e. the Province of Varese (790,000 inhabitants) and the City of Torino (1,150,000 inhabitants) in Italy, the Provinces of Navarra (520,000 inhabitants) and Zaragoza (800,000 inhabitants) in Spain, the Canton of Geneva (340,000 inhabitants) in Switzerland, and the Department of Calvados (560,000 inhabitants) in France. In all six regions, the aim was to recruit all cases, by ensuring close collaboration with hospital centers and individual otolaryngologists. In Geneva, the recruitment rate exceeded 95%; in all other centers, this rate was about 75%. The Gustave-Roussy Institute in Villejuif, France, participated in the clinical part of the study.

Clinical data have been collected on the basis of a standardized descriptive protocol made up of 86 parameters and anatomical diagrams. The clinical questionnaire mainly covered the nature of initial and prevalent symptoms, their duration, the detailed description of anatomical regions invaded by the tumor, the mobility of the vocal cords, the methods of investigation used to determine tumoral extension, lymph node involvement, distant metastases and histological diagnosis. Clinical data were collected by trained otolaryngologists after a clinical, endoscopic, radiological check-up and after an anatomicopathological test of surgical specimens of operated cases. The data on risk factors, in particular tobacco and alcohol, as well as data on sociodemographic type, were collected in an interview, the principles and methods of which have been described elsewhere [13].

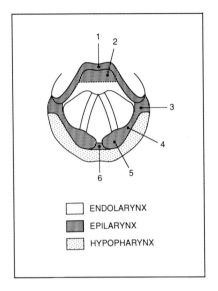

Fig. 1. The three anatomical sites of the study are: the endolarynx, the epilarynx and the hypopharynx. The epilarynx includes: (1) the epiglottis-free border; (2) the posterior surface of suprahyoid epiglottis; (3) the junction of the three folds (composed of the junction of the lateral glossoepiglottic fold, the pharyngoepiglottic fold and the aryepiglottic fold); (4) the aryepiglottic fold; (5) the arytenoid, and (6) the interarytenoid incisure [6, 11].

The classification adopted for the laryngopharyngeal region (fig. 1) includes three mains sites (endolarynx, epilarynx and hypopharynx) and nine subsites as described in a previous paper [11], where details on codes and corresponding positions in ICD-9 and ICD-0 are also provided.

All clinical questionnaires were checked, interpreted and coded by the same otolaryngologist (W.L.) who also determined the origin of the primary tumor. In 24 cases (1.8%), the site of origin could not be attributed to either of the three main sites because of extensive tumoral spread. The reliability of the assessment of tumoral origin has been evaluated by a blind counter test carried out by two other ENT specialists from a sample of 30 cases. The reproducibility proved to be excellent with regard to distribution according to the three main sites, showing minor differences at the subsite level in 4 cases only.

On the whole, 1,474 clinical questionnaires were collected and analyzed. A number was excluded from the study on the following grounds: inappropriate site of origin (47 cases); no histological confirmation (49 cases), and incomplete clinical questionnaires (11 cases). 1,374 carcinomas were analyzed, i.e. 1,367 patients, of which 7 had a double simultaneous primary site of the laryngopharynx. Controls have been randomly selected within each resident population of the six regions, according to a sampling design varying between regions [13].

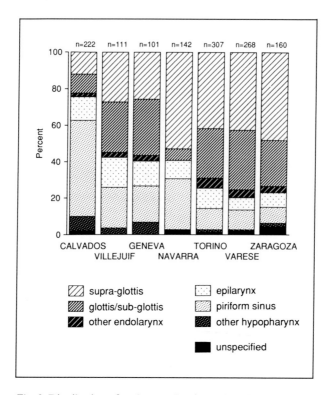

Fig. 2. Distribution of male cases by site and study center.

Results

Out of the 1,374 cancer cases studied, 1,311 were male and 63 (4.7%) were female. Regarding males, the mean age of cases is 59.7 and is not significantly different between sites. The distribution of cases by site shows an excess of endolaryngeal cancers (63.1%), followed by hypopharyngeal (24.3%) and epilaryngeal cancers (10.8%). With regard to the distribution of subsites, a slight excess in supraglottic (57.7%) versus glottic cancers (36.9%) can be noted for endolarynx; for hypopharynx, a large majority of tumors (87.5%) originated in the piriform sinus. Cancers of the epilarynx are mainly and equally distributed in the area between its anterior part (41.1%) and lateral part (37.7%); those of the posterior border represent 5% of cases. A reclassification of epilaryngeal cancers according to ICD-0

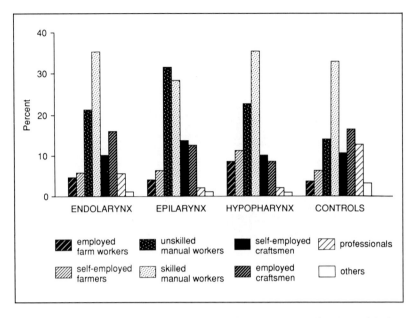

Fig. 3. Distribution of male cases and controls by site, according to social class (Villejuif excluded).

shows that about two-thirds are usually classified in the oropharynx (code 146), while only one-third are attributed to larynx (code 161) and hardly more than 10% to hypopharynx (code 148). The distribution of tumor sites by study center show considerable differences (fig. 2). The proportion of endolarynx is about 75% in Torino, Varese and Zaragoza; 60% in Navarra, Geneva and Villejuif, and 25% in Calvados. In contrast, that of hypopharynx represents only 15% in Torino, Varese and Zaragoza; 25% in Navarra, Geneva and Villejuif, and over 60% in Calvados. The proportion of epilaryngeal cancers varies slightly between centers (7–16%). Supraglottic cancers represent more than 40% of all sites in Italy and Spain; in Navarra, they exceed 50%. Their proportion is significantly lower in Geneva and in the French centers. The age-adjusted distribution of cases and controls by social class (excluding Villejuif) is shown in figure 3. Compared with other sites, endolaryngeal cancers include a relatively high proportion of employees and professionals, and a rather low proportion of unskilled manual workers and farmers. The reverse is true for hypopharyngeal cases, which include a particularly high proportion of farmers. Epilaryngeal cases tend

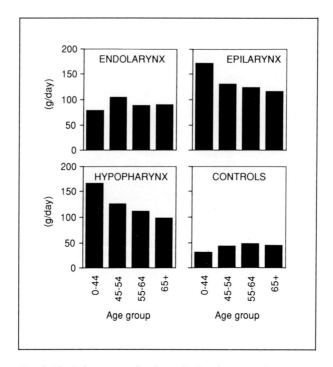

Fig. 4. Alcohol consumption in males by site, according to age.

to concentrate among unskilled manual workers. Compared with controls, cases include more unskilled manual workers and less professionals. The distribution of marital status (not shown) does not differ significantly, either between cases or between cases and controls. The mean levels of alcohol consumption vary according to site and age (fig. 4). They are significantly higher for hypopharynx and epilarynx than for endolarynx. Except for this latter site, they tend to decrease with age at diagnosis, the mean consumption level of cases diagnosed after age 65 being notably lower than that of cases diagnosed before 45. No such feature can be noted among controls. On the other hand, the mean tobacco consumption is about the same for the three sites under study, more than twice that observed in controls (fig. 5). This difference mainly results from the almost complete absence of nonsmokers among cases (between 1.8 and 3.1%, according to site), while the latter represents nearly 23.7% among controls of the same age. The increase in cancer risk related to alcohol and tobacco

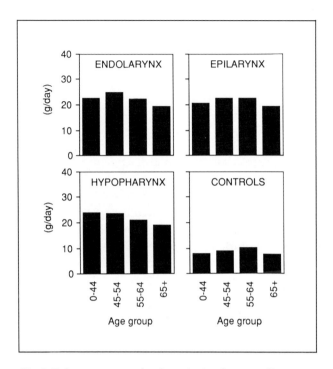

Fig. 5. Tobacco consumption in males by site, according to age.

consumption has been calculated for different levels [11]. For similar alcohol consumption, the effects of tobacco do not show statistically significant differences between sites. In contrast, when adjusted for tobacco consumption, heavy alcohol consumption entails a higher risk of getting a cancer of the epilarynx and hypopharynx than of the endolarynx, either subglottic or glottic. Relative to light drinkers (< 20 g/day), it was found that the risk associated with heavy alcohol consumption (> 120 g/day) is multiplied by 2–3 for endolarynx, and by 10–12 for epilarynx and hypopharynx. The combined effect is consistent with a multiplicative model [14]. As a consequence for this latter site, the risk associated with heavy exposure to the two factors was 140 times greater than that associated with no to moderate exposure [11]. Cancer of the laryngopharyngeal region is extremely rare among women. In our study, female cases were found mainly in the more urban and industrialized regions of Geneva, Torino and Varese. The sex ratio by site is 16:1 for endolarynx, 18:1 for epilarynx and 64:1 for hypopharynx. In addition, the high proportion of endolarynx suggests that tobacco consumption plays the major role (table 1). Endolaryngeal cases are evenly distributed between glottic and supraglottic areas, while supraglottic lesions prevail in males.

Discussion

To our knowledge, no previous case-control epidemiological study has analyzed the individual effects of alcohol and tobacco on the laryngopharynx, while also considering the epilarynx separately.

In our study, cancers of the endolarynx, epilarynx and hypopharynx account for 63%, 11% and 24%, respectively, of all laryngopharyngeal cancers in males. This distribution is, however, different between centers. In particular, the proportion of hypopharyngeal cancer is much greater in Calvados, and this of supraglottic cancer is greater in Spain and Italy. Such epidemiological studies deal with methodological problems in particular obtaining clinical information needed to determine the site of origin of the tumor. These problems are rarely discussed in the literature devoted to etiology. For both incidence and mortality data, the quality of published epidemiological data depends mainly on the accuracy of coding. Methodological studies show that the reliability of cancer mortality statistics depends on the site of the tumor. Cancers of certain organs seem to be more attractive for the coder, at least when a vague diagnosis is made by the physician filling in the death certificate [15]. No doubt these remarks

Table 1. Distribution of cases by site and study center (women)

	n	Torino	Varese	Calvados	Villejuif	Navarra	Zaragoza	Geneva
Endolarynx	50	19	12	1	3	1	1	13
Supraglottis	22	9	5	1	1	–	–	6
Glottis/subglottis	25	8	7	–	2	1	1	6
Unspecified	3	2	–	–	–	–	–	1
Epilarynx	8	4	–	–	1	–	1	2
Hypopharynx	5	1	2	–	1	–	1	–
Piriform sinus	4	1	1	–	1	–	1	–
Total	63	24	14	1	5	1	3	15

remain partly valid for incident cases recorded by cancer registries. The complexity of the laryngopharyngeal tract anatomy suggests that the corresponding subsites of cancer may be prone to miscoding, a fact which has also been mentioned in other studies [10, 16]. Knowledge of modalities of tumoral invasion [17–21], presence of anatomic barriers and concentration of lymphatic vessels is relevant to perform conservative surgery and to assess the tumoral origin. Comparison of our results with published epidemiological data suggests that the frequency of hypopharyngeal cancers can be underestimated and that of laryngeal cancers overestimated. The comparison of alcohol and tobacco consumption between cases and controls confirms the leading role of these two factors in the onset of the cancers under study. Among heavy smokers (> 26 g/day) and heavy alcohol drinkers (> 120 g/day), nearly all observed cancers are due to these excesses. Even a moderate consumption substantially increases the probability of a cancer. From our results, more than 80% of endolaryngeal cancers and more than 90% of hypopharyngeal or epilaryngeal cancers, in people smoking 8–15 g/day and also drinking 40–80 g alcohol/day, result from this double exposure. The risk caused by cigarettes could be substantially reduced by the use of filters or by not inhaling; the latter factor, however, does not significantly modify the risk for hypopharynx. The use of black tobacco, on the other hand, doubles the risk for all sites [11].

In the regions studied, farmers are characterized by a relatively low tobacco consumption, but a higher alcohol consumption; middle classes, on the other hand (employees and skilled manual workers), include more smokers who consume less alcohol [22, 23]. These observations, which more or less reflect the prevalent situation 10 years ago in most South-Western European countries, are consistent with the differences in distribution by social class within sites. Distribution by circumstances, both tobacco and alcohol consumption, as well as by socioeconomic group, shows that hypopharyngeal cancers tend to include a higher proportion of farmers and a lower proportion of employees and professionals, and that the reverse is true for endolaryngeal cancers; epilarynx cancers come in between. Our analyses of risk related to alcohol consumption on a large number of cases have not shown any difference between supraglottic and glottic sites. This result differs to several previous studies [2, 10, 24, 25, 28], and could be explained by the inclusion of a number of epilaryngeal cases – often heavier drinkers – among the supraglottic cancers under study. Ledermann [26] insisted that the epilarynx, surrounded by the alimentary 'grooves' and salivary 'reservoirs', were in permanent contact with ingested solids and liquids, while the endolarynx was protected during swallowing. From a clinical point of view, epilarynx should be considered as an independent anatomic entity, with regard to lymph node involvement, as well as therapy and prognosis [6–8, 27]. The same distinction must be made on etiological grounds. It is therefore desirable that clinicians and epidemiologists agree on the required adjustments to CIM, ICD-0 and TNM classifications.

Risk factors mainly relate to male behavior. It is therefore not surprising that the relative frequency of female cases is still very low. Reviewing the literature, the present series of female cases (n = 63) is not less significant. It shows, inter alia, that the usually observed prevalence of supraglottic cases over glottic cases cannot automatically be found among females [10]. In contrast, the mean age for female cases is about the same as for males. The mean age for cases of both sexes is not higher for glottic than for supraglottic cancer, as opposed to other observations [28]. Our analyses have demonstrated the extent of variations in mean levels of alcohol consumption according to age at diagnosis. For epilarynx and hypopharynx in particular, older cases are characterized by a much lower consumption. This may be interpreted as an indication of carcinogenesis accelerated by exposure dose: the higher it is, the quicker the lesion appears. The parallel trend is less marked for tobacco consumption. This double statement could reflect different latent periods for the risk factors, supporting the hypothesis that tobacco acts in the long term as an initiating factor, while alcohol acts in the short term as a promoting factor.

Acknowledgements

The project was partly supported by funds provided by the National Institute for Research on Alcohol Abuse and Alcoholism, USA (ADM 281-77-0026) and partly by: (a) City of Torino: Progetto finalizzato 'Oncologia' (Italian National Research Council); (b) Associazione Italiana per la Ricerca sul Cancro, Milano; (c) Consorzio per il Sistema Informativo, CSI Piemonte, Torino; (d) Province of Varese: CNR 'Progetto finalizzato Oncologia', and (e) Geneva: Swiss National Fund for Scientific Research (No. 3.809.0.79), Swiss League Against Cancer (No. 160.AK79).

The work of the following otolaryngologists and head and neck surgeons was greatly appreciated: (a) Caen: D. De Raucourt, J.P. Rame; (b) Province of Navarra: J.A. Beortlegui, R. Garcia-Tapia, J.J. Gortari, V. Martinez Lizarraga, J. Medina, J.R. Mozota, R. Rebello; (c) City of Torino: E. Amasio, R. Avataneo, S. Aversa, G. Belforte, M. Benzi, L. Bonelli, A. Brosio, F. Brunetti, G. Chiado Piat, G. Dagna, A. de Vicaris, C. Fantino, C. Italia, P. Menzio, E. Passet, A. Sartoris, G. Tabaro, W. Vitale, G. Voena; (d) Province of Varese: V. Albano, C. Cis, E. Clerici, G. Orlandi, A. Pellegrini, A. Premoli, G. Scollo, G. Spriano, L. Rovella; (e) Institut Gustave-Roussy, Villejuif: B. Luboinski, J.M. Richard, and (f) Province of Zaragoza: C. Cenjor, D. de Miguel, M. Fairen, M. Jimenez-Vergera, J.M. Marin, J. Marin Fondevila, A. Ortiz.

References

1   Muir C, Waterhouse J, Mack T, Powell J, Whelan S: Cancer Incidence in Five Continents. IARC Sci Publ No 88. Lyon, International Agency for Research on Cancer, 1987, vol V.

2   Schottenfeld D, Gantt RC, Wynder EL: The role of alcohol and tobacco in multiple primary cancers of the upper digestive systems, larynx and lung: A prospective study. Prev Med 1974;3:277–293.

3   International Classification of Diseases, rev 9. Geneva, World Health Organization, 1977.

4   International Union against Cancer (UICC): TNM Classification of Malignant Tumors, ed 4. 1987:19–26.

5   American Joint Committee on Cancer: Manual for Staging of Cancer, ed 2. Philadelphia, Lippincott, 1983. pp 25–59.

6   Guerrier Y, Pinel J, Cachin Y, Laccourreye H, Dejean Y: La chirurgie conservatrice dans le traitement des cancers du vestibule laryngé et du sinus piriforme. Paris, Arnette, 1972.

7   Laccourreye H, Brasnu D, Beutter P, Bodard M: Les épithéliomas de la margelle laryngée – Définition, classification, extension. Ann Oto-Laryngol (Paris) 1980;97: 963–976.

8   Cachin Y: Cancers du pharynx et du larynx. Facteurs diététiques. Gaz Méd France 1980;87:2845–2855.

9   Rothman JJ, Keller AZ: The effect of joint exposure to alcohol and tobacco on risk of cancer of the mouth and pharynx. J Chronic Dis 1972;25:711–716.

10 Wynder EL, Covey LS, Mabuchi K, Mushhinski M: Environmental factors in cancer of the larynx. A second look. Cancer 1976;38:1591–1601.

11 Tuyns AJ, Estève J, Raymond L, Berrino E, Benhamou E, Blanchet F, Boffetta P, Crosignani P, Del Moral A, Lehmann W, Merletti F, Péquignot G, Riboli E, Sancho-Garnier H, Terracini B, Zubiri A, Zubiri L: Cancer of the larynx/hypopharynx, tobacco and alcohol: IARC international case-control study in Turin and Varese (Italy), Zaragoza and Navarra (Spain), Geneva (Switzerland) and Calvados (France). Int J Cancer 1988;41:483–491.

12 Estève J, Péquignot G, Riboli E, Lehmann W, Merletti F, Crosignani P, Ascunce N, Zubiri L, Blanchet F, Raymond L, Repetto F, Tuyns A: Cancer of the larynx/hypopharynx and diet: A IARC international case-control study in South-Western Europe. Am J Epidemiol; in press.

13 Riboli E, Péquignot G, Repetto F, Axerio M, Raymond L, Boffetta P, Zubiri A, Del Moral A, Estève J, Tuyns AJ: A comparative study of smoking, drinking and dietary habits in population samples in France, Italy, Spain and Switzerland. I. Study design and dietary habits. Rev Epidémiol Santé Publ 1988;36:151–165.

14   Estève J, Tuyns A: Models for combined action of alcohol and tobacco on risk of cancer: What do we really know from epidemiological studies? In Feo F, Pani P, Columbano A, Garcea R (eds): Chemical Carcinogenesis. New York, Plenum Publishing, 1988.
15   Percy C, Dolman A: Comparison of the coding of death certificates related to cancer in seven countries. Public Health Rep 1978;93:335–350.
16   Till JE, Bruce WR, Elwau A, Till MJ, Niederer J, Reid J, Hawkins NV, Rider WD: A preliminary analysis of end results for cancer of the larynx. Laryngoscope 1975;85:259–275.
17   Tucker GF: Human larynx coronal section atlas. Washington, Armed Forces Institute of Pathology, 1971.
18   Micheau C, Luboinski B, Sancho H, Cachin Y: Modes of invasion of cancer of the larynx. A statistical, histological, and radioclinical analysis of 120 cases. Cancer 1976;38:346–360.
19   Harrison DFN: Pathology of hypopharyngeal cancer in relation to surgical management. J Laryngol Otolaryngol 1970;84:349–366.
20   Kirchner JA: Pyriform sinus cancer: A clinical and laboratory study. Ann Otolaryngol 1975;84:793–804.
21   Olofsson J, Van Norstrand AWP: Growth and spread of laryngeal and hypopharyngeal carcinoma with reflections on the effect of preoperative irradiation. Acta Otolaryngol (Stockh) 1973;308(suppl):7–84.
22   Péquignot G, Crosignani P, Terracini B, Ascunce N, Zubiri A, Raymond L, Estève J, Tuyns AJ: A comparative study of smoking, drinking and dietary habits in population samples in France, Italy, Spain and Switzerland. III. Study design and dietary habits. Rev Epidémiol Santé Publ 1988;36:151–165.
23   Berrino F, Merletti F, Zubiri A, Del Moral A, Raymond L, Estève J, Tuyns AJ: A comparative study of smoking, drinking and dietary habits in population samples in France, Italy, Spain and Switzerland. II. Tobacco smoking. Rev Epidémiol Santé Publ 1988;36:166–176.
24   Elwood JM, Pearson JCG, Skippen DH, Jackson SM: Alcohol, smoking, social and occupational factors in the aetiology of cancer of the oral cavity, pharynx and larynx. Int J Cancer 1984;34:603–612.
25   Brugère J, Guenel P, Leclerc A, Rodriguez J: Differential effects of tobacco and alcohol in cancer of the larynx, pharynx and mouth. Cancer 1986;57:391–395.
26   Ledermann M: The anatomy of cancer with special reference to tumors of the upper air and food passages. J Laryngol Otolaryngol 1964;78:181–211.
27   Brasnu D, Lacau St Gilly J, Laccourreye H: Cancers de la margelle laryngée; in Brugère J (ed): Cancers des voies aérodigestives supérieures. Paris, Flammarion, 1987, pp 281–292.
28   Kleinsasser O: Epidemiologie, Ätiologie und Pathogenese; in Tumoren des Larynx und des Hypopharynx. Stuttgart, Thieme, 1987, pp 2–25.

W. Lehmann, MD, Clinic of Otorhinolaryngology, Cantonal University Hospital, 24, rue Micheli-du-Crest, CH–1211 Geneva 4 (Switzerland)

Pfaltz CR, Arnold W, Kleinsasser O (eds): Bearing of Basic Research on Clinical
Otolaryngology. Adv Otorhinolaryngol. Basel, Karger, 1991, vol 46, pp 157–164

Variations in Histopathogenesis of Squamous Cell Carcinoma of the Upper Aerodigestive Tract

O. Kleinsasser

HNO-Klinik der Philipps-Universität, Marburg, FRG

Tumors of the vocal cords often cause functional impairment, result-ing in a hoarseness, even if they are only a few millimeters in size. Like in no other inner organ, laryngologists and pathologists have the possibility to study the clinical and microscopical picture of precursors and early stages of squamous cell carcinomas and to follow the changes within the epithe-lium from precancerosis via preinvasive to minimally invasive or already macroinvasive stages of cancerogenesis. (It should be mentioned that changes similar to those on the vocal cords are seen in all other regions of the upper aerodigestive tract – but here early stages are observed relatively rarely.)

Based on the fundamental studies of gynecologists and pathologists, we thought for a long time that carcinoma always must develop via a precancerous stage. Histologic examination of surgical specimens however have enabled us to obtain many new insights into the details of morpho-genesis and to recognize its high variability. The classical opinion on the microscopically visible steps in cancerogenesis can be outlined as fol-lows:

In certain predilection areas within the upper aerodigestive tract nor-mal-appearing squamous epithelium becomes hyperplastic or – in rare cases – atrophic. Within this hyperplastic or atrophic epithelium cellular atypias and disturbances of differentiation arise (fig. 1). The number of atypical cells increases until finally a state of severe dysplasia is reached (fig. 2). If all layers of the epithelium consist of atypical or undifferentiated

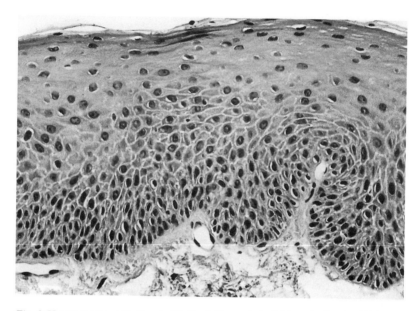

Fig. 1. Hyperplastic epithelium with single hyperchromatic nuclei in the lower and middle layers.

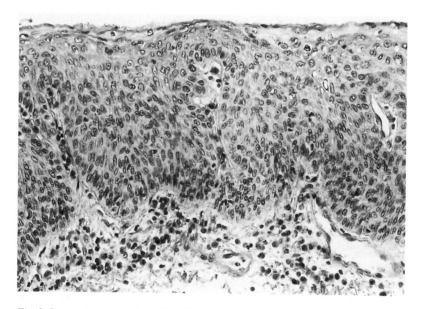

Fig. 2. Severe dysplasia of vocal cord epithelium.

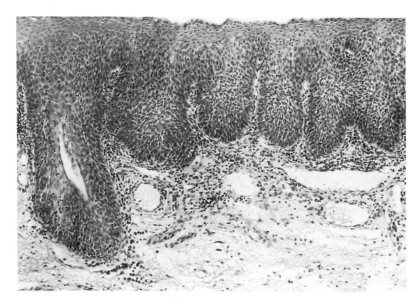

Fig. 3. Classical carcinoma in situ of the vocal cord. The whole epithelium consists of immature nuclei.

cells the lesion is called carcinoma in situ (fig. 3). In my opinion there is no fundamental or biologic difference between carcinoma in situ and severe epithelial dysplasia as both lesions are only variations in differentiation during the preinvasive stage and both finally proceed to an infiltrating squamous cell carcinoma via a microinvasive stage.

However, there is also another possibility: The first visible lesion may be a sharply circumscribed *tumor* surrounded by normal-appearing epithelium. Most of these lesions have an irregular surface with verrucous, cauliflower like or even thorn-like papillary projections. They are therefore called keratosis, senile papilloma, verruca, etc. These lesions are true tumors from the beginning. Microscopically some of them show no atypical cells – they behave like benign tumors and stay benign in the majority of cases and we call them benign keratomas (fig. 4) – this is the benign counterpart of squamous cell carcinoma. Many others however mainly consist of atypical cells but without infiltrating growth. These tumors are true precanceroses and they finally will proceed to infiltrating carcinomas. Nobody can say how long it will take until these precancerous tumors turn into true cancers.

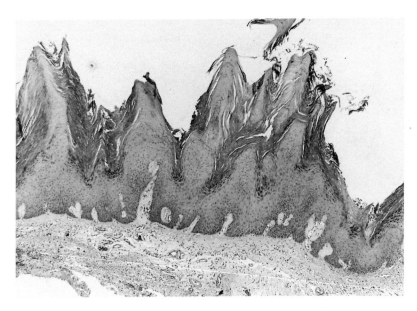

Fig. 4. Verrucous benign keratoma of a vocal cord, no atypical cells.

This means that the histological picture of carcinoma in situ can be a rapidly progressing early intraepithelial stage, of a continually developing carcinoma where infiltration could develop even within a few days. A morphologically completely identical lesion however may remain unchanged for many years before it becomes malignant like, for example, Bowen's disease. One could postulate that the latter, the true precancerous tumors, are 'restrained carcinomas' whose growth is inhibited for a long time by immunologic factors.

Like there are two different ways in the development of carcinoma, carcinomata in situ themselves also grow differently. Observation of the marginal zone of a carcinoma in situ shows that the tumor can develop distinct sharp borders to the neighboring epithelium. This border can be vertical or wedge-like, giving the impression that the tumor cells at the advancing edge lift up the neighboring epithelium like a plowshare, sliding along the basal membrane even into the excretory ducts of the mucosal glands and carpeting them. This suggests that the carcinoma in situ grows interstitially by division of its own cells.

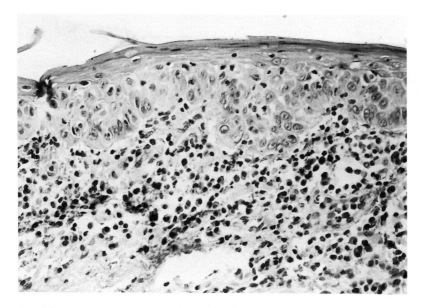

Fig. 5. In areas surrounding a carcinoma in situ the basal cells show severe atypias suggesting an appositional growth of the tumor.

In many other cases one can see a successive transition from a central carcinoma in situ to an epithelium with a decreasing number of aypias toward the periphery. These cases demonstrate an appositional growth: more and more basal cells from the surrounding area are incorporated into the growth of the carcinoma in situ. The pathologist Herwig Hamperl called this process an 'infectious growth' (fig. 5). It is obvious that it is much easier to completely remove a circumscribed lesion with pushing borders than a diffusely extending carcinoma in situ with broad paracancerous zones of dysplastic epithelium, without sharp delineation.

Unfortunately until today microscopical investigations do not allow to differentiate between the carcinomata in situ which are short intraepithelial stages in the process of cancerogenesis and those that are true precancerous lesions which will take maybe years until they proceed to an infiltrating tumor.

The way from a carcinoma in situ to an infiltrating carcinoma can be followed by studying microcarcinomas. Infiltrating carcinomas are often still surrounded by the remnants of carcinoma in situ (fig. 6). This zone has

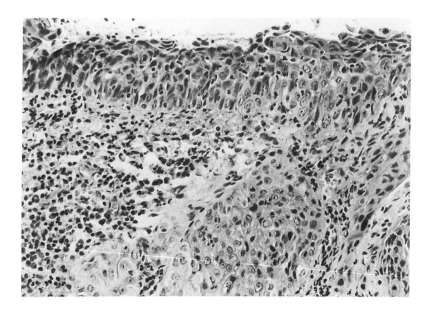

Fig. 6. Carcinomatous 'Randbelag' corresponding to a carcinoma in situ around the infiltrating tumor.

been called the 'Randbelag'. The infiltrating carcinoma usually lies in the center of this epithelial field, but may be excentric. Several infiltrating foci of cancer may exist. Systematic investigations have shown that a Randbelag can be found in 30–40% of all laryngeal cancers, especially in the non-keratinizing varieties. The fact that a new infiltrating carcinoma may arise from these remnants of the Randbelag is of practical significance.

Investigations by serial sections of surgical specimens, however, have shown that classical carcinoma in situ is in no way an obligatory precursor of invasive carcinoma or that a precancerous lesion must not always proceed the development of cancer. This means that the long nourished theory that all squamous cell carcinomas could be diagnosed in a very early preinvasive state, if only we were attentive enough, is wrong. Many squamous cell cancers arise from simple hyperplastic squamous epithelium or even atrophic epithelium, with little or no atypia in the middle and upper cell layers (fig. 7). In these cases invasion into the depth starts directly from the basal cells, without any alteration of the surface – an early diagnosis by endoscopy is impossible since the carcinoma is hidden by a layer of nor-

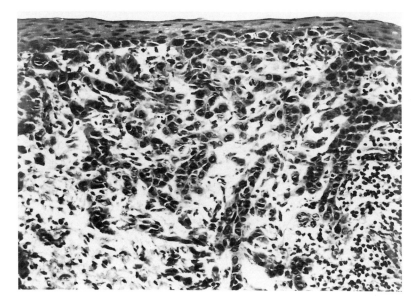

Fig. 7. Infiltrating, highly malignant carcinoma arising from the basal layers of an atrophic epithelium.

mal-appearing epithelium, until exulceration of the surface indicates underlying infiltrating growth.

Many squamous cell carcinomas arise from a relatively small area and spread into the depth like the roots of a tree. The extent of this area is of great significance for the selection of therapy. In addition to these unicentrical and circumscribed cancers, extensive layers of severely atypical epithelium covering large surfaces (for instance both vocal folds or extensive parts of the buccal mucosa) can be observed. They obviously spread like a drop of oil on water. Areas of in situ carcinoma alternate with sections of microinvasive carcinoma and confluent foci of macroinvasive carcinoma. These tumors which are the result of field cancerization are called carpet carcinomas or superficial spreading carcinomas. We observe them relatively often in up to about 20% of all cases in the upper aerodigestive tract. They are difficult to treat since they are less suitable for surgery and often do not respond well to radiotherapy. Primary multiple carcinomas, i.e. individually infiltrating lesions separated from each other by a zone of normal-appearing epithelium, can be considered as variations of these carpet tumors.

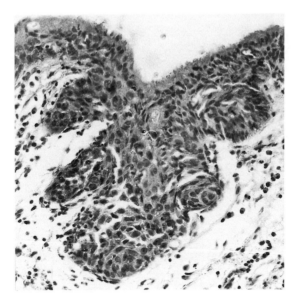

Fig. 8. Squamous cell carcinoma arising from cylindrical respiratory epithelium in the subglottic area of the larynx.

Finally I have to mention that for a long time we thought that squamous cell carcinoma always arises from either original squamous epithelium or from squamous epithelium developed by squamous metaplasia. Now we have seen a few cases where in the neighborhood of a squamous cell carcimoma the basal cells of cylindrical ciliated respiratory epithelium started to develop carcinomatous outgrowths as well (fig. 8). All these histopathologic variations in cancerogenesis may be considered to be interesting mainly for the lover of histopathology. However, they have practical importance since they give us insights into and understanding of the growth and spread of squamous cell carcinoma of the upper aerodigestive tract and help us to select an optimal therapy tailored to the individual case.

Prof. Dr. O. Kleinsasser, HNO-Klinik der Philipps-Universität, Deutschhausstrasse 3, D-W–3550 Marburg (FRG)

Pfaltz CR, Arnold W, Kleinsasser O (eds): Bearing of Basic Research on Clinical Otolaryngology. Adv Otorhinolaryngol. Basel, Karger, 1991, vol 46, pp 165–175

Multiple Primary Malignancies

M. Savary, Ph. Monnier, R. Pasche, E. Brossard, Ph. Pasche, F. Lang

ENT Clinic, CHUV, Lausanne, Switzerland

The existence of multiple cancers in the upper aerodigestive tract is known at least since Broca's observations in the middle of the 19th century [6]. But the statistical data collected up to now vary quite a lot depending on the time and the country they come from, the type of the study (retrospective or prospective), and especially the methodology used (clinical and postmortem data or endoscopic and cytological screening) [1–4, 7, 12, 13, 15, 17].

The aim of this publication is to put together our knowledge about the phenomenon of multiple tumors arising in the upper aerodigestive tract, in the light of 27 years' experience with oncological endoscopy, taking into account clinical, endoscopic and histological data. The place of panendoscopy is discussed.

Material and Method

This paper reviews the results of four oncological studies which took place at the ENT Clinic of the University Hospital in Lausanne, Switzerland. The first is a retrospective study of 1,091 patients with carcinomas of mouth, pharynx and larynx treated between 1967 and 1982 [15]. The three others are prospective trials. From 1984 on, we introduced a standard diagnostic and surveillance procedure for ENT cancer patients (fig. 1). The panendoscopy takes place at two definite moments in this procedure – first, during the pretherapeutic evaluation, and second, during the control evaluation 2 years after treatment. We call 'panendoscopy' a complete examination of the airways and the upper digestive tract that takes place in two steps: for the mouth, the pharynx and the larynx, we use a wall-fixed surgical microscope with a laryngeal mirror or the Von Stuckrad laryngoscope. For the esophagus, the trachea and the bronchi, we use both rigid and fiberoptic endoscopes under general anesthesia [2, 8, 15–17].

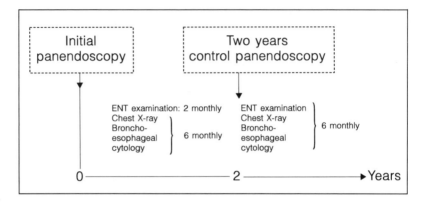

Fig. 1. Standard diagnostic and surveillance procedure for ENT cancer patients.

Vital staining with toluidine blue is systematically applied in the flat surface of the digestive mucosa in the mouth, the pharynx and the esophagus [10, 16, 17]. Because of its affinity with cell nuclei, toluidine blue will stain the areas of severe dysplasia or of carcinoma. In this way, the tumor limits can be determined accurately and the satellite lesions detected [10]. This vital staining was introduced because in the hypopharynx and the esophagus, early cancers take most of the time the form of flat and red discolorations which are hard to make out by simple macroscopic inspection [8, 9, 11, 17].

In order to check for the usefulness of this type of oncological panendoscopy in the pretherapeutic evaluation of patients, we have collected 100 successive pretherapeutic panendoscopies in patients with cancers of the mouth, pharynx or larynx, from 1984 to 1986 [2]. In a similar way, we have evaluated the yield of the control panendoscopy systematically done 2 years after treatment of the primary cancer by collecting the results of another 100 consecutive control panendoscopies, from 1988 to 1989.

The third prospective study is a morphological study of 190 early cancers, evaluating and comparing macroscopic, endoscopic and histologic appearance of early cancers in the upper digestive tract (mouth, pharynx and esophagus) [8].

Results

Retrospective Study

According to the classical oncological definition of second primary cancers given by Warren and Gates [20] in 1932, we have realized in 1984 a first retrospective study concerning a group of 1,091 patients with ENT cancers [15]. This study records 180 patients (16.5%) with either synchronous or metachronous multiple malignancies, adding up to a total of 236 second primary tumors (table 1). Fifty-three of these second tumors are

Table 1. Occurrence rate of second primary cancers (SPCs) in the upper digestive and lower respiratory tract

ENT primary cancers		1,091 = 100%
Patients with	SPCs	180 = 16.5%
	simultaneous SPCs	92 = 8.4%
	successive SPCs	88 = 8.1%
Patients with	1 SPC	142 = 142
	2 SPCs	26 = 52
	3 SPCs	8 = 24
	4 SPCs	2 = 8
	5 SPCs	2 = 10
		236 tumors

Table 2. Buccopharyngeal cancer: occurrence rate of second primary cancers (synchronous and metachronous)

		n	%
Patients with	primary buccopharyngeal cancer	795	100
	second primary cancers	146	18.5

located in the ENT region, 23% in the esophagus and 24% in the bronchi [15].

The location of the second tumor in relationship to the site of the primary tumor is as follows: (1) when the primary tumor is found in the buccopharyngeal region, the prevalence of second primary tumors is 18.5% (table 2) and 82% of these second tumors are located in the *upper digestive tract* (table 3), and (2) when the primary tumor is in the larynx, the prevalence of second tumors is much lower (11.5%) (table 4). It is interesting to point out that 45% of these second tumors are not located in the airways but in the *upper digestive tract* (table 5).

If we compare the anatomical site of these second tumors and their time of development (synchronous/metachronous), we notice that most esophageal second primaries (28/45) are diagnosed simultaneously, while most bronchial second cancers (31/45) arise later on [15]. The 5-year cumulative risk for a second tumor, when calculated in an actuarial way,

Table 3. Buccopharyngeal cancer: location of second primary cancers (198 SPCs found in 146 patients)

Location	n	%	
Mouth and pharynx	120	61	} 82% upper digestive tract
Esophagus	42	21	
Larynx	10	5	} 18% lower respiratory tract
Bronchi	26	13	
Total	198	100	

Table 4. Laryngeal cancer: occurrence rate of second primary cancer (synchronous and metachronous)

		n	%
Patient with	primary laryngeal cancer	296	100
	second primary cancers	34	11.5

Table 5. Laryngeal cancer: location of second primary cancers (38 SPCs found in 34 patients

Location	n	%	
Mouth and pharynx	14	37	} 45% upper digestive tract
Esophagus	3	8	
Larynx	2	5	} 55% lower respiratory tract
Bronchi	19	50	
Total	38	100	

that means exclusively for patients really exposed to the risk (heavy drinkers *and* smokers), added up to 32% for the group of patients followed up between 1976 and 1982. The 5-year cumulative risk for a third tumor in patients with already two tumors rises up to 55% [15]. This study extends over a long period of time (15 years) and is characterized by the change of

Table 6. Prevalence of synchronous second primary cancers

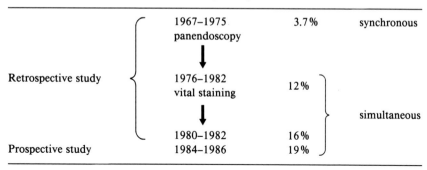

Retrospective study	1967–1975 panendoscopy	3.7%	synchronous
	1976–1982 vital staining	12%	simultaneous
	1980–1982	16%	
Prospective study	1984–1986	19%	

Table 7. Value of the initial panendoscopy in ENT cancer patients (n = 100)

Second primary cancers	Patients	Tumors
1 SPC	13	13
2 SPCs	3	6
3 SPCs	3	9
Total yield	19 (19%)	28 (28%)

methodology used to discover second tumors (table 6). From 1967 to 1975, systematic screening for a second cancer was not applied. In 1976, we introduced the systematic pretherapeutic panendoscopy and in 1980, the use of vital staining with toluidine blue. This resulted in a dramatic increase of the diagnosis of synchronous and simultaneous second primary cancers. This increase seems to be directly related to the decrease in the prevalence of successive second tumors during the first year following treatment [15].

Prospective Studies

The prospective study number 1, evaluating 100 successive pretherapeutic panendoscopies, points out that 19 patients out of 100 show a second cancer with a total of 28 simultaneous second primary tumors (table 7). Twelve of these are located in the ENT region, 10 in the esophagus and 6 in the bronchi (table 8). In 89% of the cases, the second tumor is staged as an in situ carcinoma or T_1 carcinoma (table 9). Sixteen times out

Table 8. Location of simultaneous second primaries in ENT cancer patients[1]

Location of primary cancer		Location of second primary tumors		
		ENT	esophagus	bronchi
Buccopharynx	77	10	10	3
Larynx	23	2	–	3
Total	100	12	10	6

bronchoesophagoscopy

[1] 58% of these second cancers could only be discovered at bronchoesophagoscopy.

Table 9. Staging of the simultaneous second primary cancers (n = 28) in ENT cancer patients

Localization/staging	ENT	Esophagus	Bronchi	
T_{is}	4	2	3	} 89%
T_1	7	6	3	
T_2	1	2	–	
T_3	–	–	–	

of 19, the therapeutic program had to be modified following the panendoscopy [2].

In a similar way, our prospective study number 2 checks for the yield of 100 successive panendoscopies systematically done 2 years after treatment of the primary cancer. Seventy-eight patients were asymptomatic, showed no visible lesions at ENT examination and at chest X-ray, and had a negative bronchoesophageal cytology.

For the remaining 22 patients, one or more of these data were positive. Twenty-one percent of the patients showed one or several malignant lesions, with a total of 29 malignancies (table 10). Nineteen were second cancers and 10 were recurrences. Eleven second primaries were located in the ENT region, 5 in the esophagus and 3 in the bronchi (table 11). In 94% of the cases, the second tumor was staged as an in situ or a T_1 carcinoma,

Table 10. Value of 2 years' control panendoscopy in patients previously treated for ENT cancer (n = 100)

	Patients	Lesions
Recurrences only	6	7
Recurrences + second primaries	2	7
Second primary tumors only	13	15
Total	21 (21%)	29 (29%)

Table 11. Location of metachronous second primary cancers in ENT cancer patients[1]

Location	Discovered at		Total
	ENT exam	bronchoesophagoscopy	
Mouth and oropharynx	3	4	7
Hypopharynx	–	4	4
Larynx	–	–	–
Bronchi	–	3	3
Esophagus	–	5	5
Total	3	16	19

[1] 42% of these second cancers could only be discovered at bronchoesophagoscopy.

the large majority being in situ cancers (table 12). But the most important fact is that, in the group of 78 asymptomatic patients without any pathology at ENT examination, chest X-ray and bronchoesophageal cytology, 12 second malignancies were discovered (table 13). The yield of 2 years' control panendoscopy is therefore 21% for the number of patients and 29% for the number of malignant lesions, if we take into account the 100 successive procedures. On the other hand, when performed on patients with no symptoms and no pathology at ENT examination, chest X-ray and bronchoesophageal cytology, this control panendoscopy shows a yield of 13% for the number of patients and of 15% for the number of second tumors.

Finally, a morphological prospective study allows us to stress a peculiar aspect of tumor multifocality: it is the multifocal tendency in the local phenomenon of carcinogenesis in itself, meaning multicentric field carci-

Table 12. Staging of the metachronous second primary cancers (n = 19)

Localization/staging	ENT	Esophagus	Bronchi	
T_{is}	8	4	2	
T_1	2	1	1	} 94%
T_2	1			
T_3	–			
T_4	–			

Table 13. Value of 2 years' control panendoscopy in asymptomatic patients previously treated for ENT cancer, with no pathology at ENT examination, chest X-ray and bronchoesophageal cytology (n = 78)

Recurrence	Second primaries	
	patients	lesions
ENT	4	5
Bronchi	2	3
Esophagus	4	4
Total	10 (12.6%)	12 (15.4%)

nogenesis or tumor multicentricity. This study was also made possible by the systematic use of the oncological panendoscopy done on patients with ENT cancer, leading to the diagnosis of a great number of early cancers and allowing to study their morphology in the ENT region, the esophagus and the bronchi as well. For the esophagus, the definition of early cancer is a precise one [5, 8, 11, 14, 19]. According to the UICC, it implies a carcinoma that does not invade the lamina muscularis propria and that has no associated lymph node involvement or distant metastasis [5, 19]. For the mouth and pharynx, where the lamina muscularis mucosae is absent, the definition is less precise but we can admit that early lesions should not extend further than the basal membrane [9].

In the mouth, pharynx and esophagus, the endoscopic aspect appears similar and corresponds either to an elevated white lesion, to a slightly depressed red discoloration, to a combination of both or to an absence of visible lesion where only the vital staining will make the detection possible [8–11]. The prevalence of white elements is less frequent in the esophagus than in the mouth, whereas the red discoloration appears more frequently in the esophagus than in the mouth [8].

But the most striking fact is the multicentric character of these early lesions existing in the esophagus and in the pharynx as well as in the mouth. Out of 73 early esophageal cancers, that multicentric character was present in 82% of the cases. A focal isolated tumoral lesion is rarely observed in the esophagus [8, 9, 11]. Most of the time, the endoscopy reveals that spotted zones of carcinogenesis spread on a determined segment of the esophagus. When comparing the macroscopic pattern obtained after toluidine blue staining to the histologic map obtained after serial sections of the resected specimen, one finds also histologically this multicentric aspect of the disease made by juxtaposition of various lesions at different stages, ranging from dysplasia to submucosal carcinoma [8]. That is why we cannot possibly evaluate the maximal in-depth extent of an early carcinoma by biopsy, even if many specimens are taken. So the staging of a superficial cancer of the upper digestive tract is much more difficult than it seems at first sight. However, staging of 'early' cancer should be as accurate as possible, because of the actual tendency to endoscopic treatment.

In the hypopharynx, the same multicentric aspect of early cancer is the rule [8]. Statistically, out of 16 early hypopharyngeal carcinomas, the multicentric aspect was present in 90% of the cases [9]. Thus, the morphological study of cancer of hypopharynx and esophagus in its beginning stage recalls the 'field' carcinogenesis evoked by Slaughter et al. [18] in 1953 for the oral cavity.

Conclusions

In the upper aerodigestive tract, the squamous cell carcinogenesis shows a tendency towards arising of multiple tumors that we call *multifocality*. In buccopharyngeal primary cancers, the second tumors are mainly found in the upper digestive tract (82%), while in laryngeal cancers, they are found in the respiratory as well as in the upper digestive tract, thus confirming a certain similarity of the oncological risk in the respiratory and the upper digestive tract. The 5-year cumulative risk to develop a second tumor in patients with one cancer is 1:3. The 5-year cumulative risk to develop a third tumor in patients with two cancers is 1:2.

The squamous cell carcinogenesis shows also a tendency towards simultaneous arising of multiple cancer foci within the same limited mucosal area, a phenomenon we call *multicentricity*. In the upper digestive tract, this multicentric pattern is present in 80% of early cancers. Multicentricity makes staging of early lesion difficult and careful attention should be paid to the interpretation of biopsies before choosing the adequate treatment.

The yield of the *initial panendoscopy* appears to be 19% for the number of patients and 28% for the number of second tumors. The yield of *2 years' control panendoscopy* is 21% for the number of patients and 29% for the number of second tumors. When performed in asymptomatic patients with no pathology at ENT examination, chest X-ray and bronchoesophageal cytology, the yield of 2 years' control panendoscopy is 13% for the number of patients and 15% for the number of second tumors.

With our screening program (fig. 1) the detection rate of early second cancers has improved in a significant way over the years, while in the same time the discovery of extensive second tumors has become infrequent, as well as the discovery of metachronous tumors in the first year after treatment of the primary cancer. Eighty percent of the second cancers discovered at initial or at control panendoscopy are in situ or T_1 cancers; 50% of these second cancers may not be diagnosed by an ENT control examination, because they are localized in the esophagus or the bronchi. The discovery of a second cancer at initial or at control panendoscopy modifies the treatment program in 5 cases out of 6.

Even if there is no proof that this screening program has a survival value for the patients, it represents an effort towards detection of an early lesion, which is a most promising way towards progress in oncological treatment. It also leads to a better knowledge of the natural history of upper aerodigestive carcinogenesis, to a better knowledge of morphology of early cancer, to progress in staging early malignant lesions and to progress in nonmutilating therapeutic means of early cancer, like photodynamic treatment or immunomodulators.

References

1   Andrieu-Guitrancourt, J.; Brossard-Legrand, M.; Happich, J.L.; Lamy, J.M.: Endoscopie systématique de l'œsophage au cours des cancers buccaux, pharyngés et laryngés. Annls Oto-lar., Paris *92:* 659–666 (1975).
2   Brossard, E.; Savary, M.; Monnier, Ph.: Cancers bucco-pharyngo-laryngés: bilan des 100 dernières pan-endoscopies pré-thérapeutiques; in Kellerhals, B., et al.: ORL –

Aktuelle Probleme der Otorhinolaryngologie, vol. 10, pp. 287–293 (Huber, Bern 1987).

3   Cachin, Y.: Cancers multiples concomitants des voies aéro-digestives supérieures. J. fr. Oto-rhino-laryngol 3: 667–689 (1972).

4   Dargent, M.; Noel, P.; Pierluca, P.: Résultats d'une étude nécropsique de la muqueuse œsophagienne chez les sujets ayant présenté des cancers de la sphère oro-pharyngolaryngée. Bull. Acad. natn. Méd 156: 408–415 (1972).

5   Endo, M.; Kobayashi, S.; Suzuki, H.; Takemoto, T.; Nakayama, K.: Diagnosis of early esophageal cancer. Endoscopy 2: 61–66 (1971).

6   Fauvet, J.; Chavy, A.; Piet, R.: Les cancers primitifs multiples. Revue Pratn 14: 2149–2174 (1964).

7   Moertel, Ch: Multiple primary malignant neoplasms, historical perspectives. Cancer 40: 1786–1792 (1977).

8   Monnier, Ph.: Le carcinome épidermoïde 'précoce' de la voie digestive supérieure; thèse Fac. Méd. Lausanne (1986).

9   Monnier, Ph.; Savary, M.; Pasche, R.: Le carcinome 'précoce' de l'hypopharynx; in Kellerhals, B., et al.: ORL – Aktuelle Probleme der Otorhinolaryngologie, vol 7, pp. 111–121 (Huber, Bern 1984).

10 Monnier, Ph., Savary, M.; Pasche, R.: Contribution of toluidine blue to bucco-pharyngo-esophageal cancerology. Acta endoscop 11: 299–315 (1981).

11 Monnier, Ph.; Savary, M.; Pasche, R.; Anani, P.: Intraepithelial carcinoma of the esophagus: endoscopic morphology. Endoscopy 13: 185–191 (1981).

12 Mounier-Kuhn, P.; Gaillard, J.; Rebattu, J.P.; Jakubowicz, B.: Statistique des cancers multiples à la clinique oto-rhino-laryngologique de Lyon de 1950 à 1962. J. fr. Oto-rhino-laryngol. 12: 627–652 (1963).

13 Panosetti, E.; Luboinski, B.; Mamelle, G.; Richard, J.M.: Multiple synchronous and metachronous cancers of the upper digestive tract: a nine-year study. Laryngoscope 99: 1267–1273 (1989).

14 Pasche, Ph.: Le staging endoscopique du cancer précoce pour la voie digestive supérieure; in Kellerhals, B., et al.: ORL – Aktuelle Probleme der Otorhinolaryngologie, vol. 12, pp. 131–137 (Huber, Bern 1989).

15 Pasche, R.; Savary, M.; Monnier, Ph.: Le risque de seconde localisation tumorale chez le porteur d'un cancer de la bouche, du pharynx ou du larynx; in Kellerhals, B., et al.: ORL – Aktuelle Probleme der Otorhinolaryngologie, vol. 7, pp. 134–142 (Huber, Bern 1984).

16 Savary, M.; Crausaz, P.H.; Monnier, Ph.: La place de l'endoscopie totale aéro-digestive supérieure en cancérologie. Schweiz. med. Wschr. 109: 838–840 (1979).

17 Savary, M.; Monnier, Ph.; Pasche, R.: Les cancers oro-pharyngo-laryngés: le bilan endoscopique. Helv. chir. Acta 50: 509–518 (1983).

18 Slaughter, P.J.; Southwick, H.W.; Smejkal, E.: 'Field cancerization' in oral stratified squamous epithelium. Clinical implications of multicentric origin. Cancer 6: 963–968 (1953).

19 TNM Classification of malignant tumors; 3rd ed. (UICC, Geneva 1979).

20 Warren, S.; Gates, O.: Multiple primary malignant tumors; a survey of the literature and a statistical study. Am. J. Cancer 16: 1358–1414 (1932).

Prof. Dr. M. Savary, ENT Clinic, CHUV, 46, rue du Bugnon,
CH-1011 Lausanne (Switzerland)

Pfaltz CR, Arnold W, Kleinsasser O (eds): Bearing of Basic Research on Clinical
Otolaryngology. Adv Otorhinolaryngol. Basel, Karger, 1991, vol 46, pp 176–179

Discussion

Kleinsasser (Marburg): Dr. de Villiers I'm sure that some of our patients are persons
full with viruses who never get a carcinoma and others have just a few and do get a
carcinoma. And Dr. Tuyns, as we all know, you can smoke 100 cigarettes a day and have a
mucosa like a virgin and never get a carcinoma, whereas others smoke only 5 cigarettes
and die from a larynx cancer. Do you have any explanations or ideas what additional
promoting factors are necessary within this range of well-known carcinogenic factors until
a cancer really develops? Dr. de Villiers, may I ask you first?

de Villiers (Heidelberg): As I showed in a model we believe that it is a multi-stage
development of a normal cell developing into a carcinomatous cell and if you think of the
different steps that have to occur before you can reach the stage of the truly malignant cell
it will probably take years. All these different steps have to occur within one cell, that
means you have to have a co-factor such as chemicals or whatever is coming from the
outside, inactivating the cellular gene which would control the action of the virus in the
cell. And of course you need the virus in the cell as well as you have to have a primary
infection of the virus into the cell and as I said we believe now that even a second step
from a premalignant lesion to a malignant lesion is necessary in that a second integration
of this viral DNA within the cellular genome occurs. So all these actions have to take place
in one cell and that is why you have these long latency periods from the primary infection
via virus until the development of a real tumour, because most of these tumours are
monoclonal.

Kleinsasser: Dr. Schroeder, what do you think about these varying latency periods?

Schroeder (Marburg): In the paper of Dr. Tuyns and Dr. Lehmann we saw this
beautiful dose-response relationship and I'm sorry to say we could not find this relationship in our series. We saw very short exposure times and short latency periods of those
patients and we saw very long periods of exposure and long latency periods and so, I think
(for the adenocarcinomas only) in our case we didn't find all those factors that are
involved with this type of cancer and we have to search for other factors, i.e. for other
co-carcinogenes and other promoting factors responsible for these differences.

Tuyns (Lyon): There is one thing that I should like to say right at the beginning:
When the topics of this session are called aetiology, epidemiology and pathogenesis, aetiology implies a concept of causes and a clear understanding of combination of cause of

agents. Now I think epidemiologists never dare speak about causes because they think that this is beyond their reach. This is why we keep talking about risk factors and these are expressed in terms of probability. Some go further than that – many of my colleague epidemiologists would stop after having discovered that a risk of tumour is increased. This is why I kept referring to relative risks and I think that some of my colleagues did the same. I think that even though this may not be completely satisfactory for our scientific mind I think it is of a great practical importance because with this concept it is emphasized that tobacco, alcohol or wood dust, as Dr. Schroeder showed, are risk factors. This has got practical indications. We know now that if we can reduce the exposure we are going to reduce the risk of getting such cases.

Kleinsasser: Allow me a further question to Dr. Jensen. You mentioned that Eskimos and Innuits in Alaska have a high incidence of malignant parotid tumours and this is the same for the Greenland Innuits. Do you know other examples of this obviously genetically induced high incidence of specific cancers?

Jensen (Copenhagen): We know it of the nasopharynx carcinoma in the Southern Chinese population. The question is really whether these tumours are genetically induced, or whether there is a genetic factor involved. Indeed that was thought for a long time to be the case for the nasopharyngeal cancer in the Chinese, but then there are these ideas of a special food being responsible. This has been around for a long time, about 4–5 years ago, and you may know from Los Angeles they reported on some very elegant studies that have been carried out in Hong Kong and in Southern California in parallel in the Chinese population and they demonstrated that the consumption of salted fish could indeed be associated with – and they carefully used the word 'associated with' for the same reason as Dr. Tuyns mentioned I am an epidemiologist – so this could be associated with an increased risk and that means an increased probability of developing this particular tumour in this population.

I should like to go back to your first question because for this cancer as well as for many other cancers I think we have expressed ourselves cautiously in the past as epidemiologists, saying that there are certainly multiple steps that the process has to take from the development of a normal cell into a malignant cell, and that some host factors play a role. That again is a very cautious way of expressing things. We know that there are various DNA repair mechanisms for instance. Among these factors now Dr. De Villier has shown with the group of Heidelberg a very elegant work demonstrating how viral factors that are present in many if not all persons actually, may be quite important in this process. These discoveries may lead us to prevention and perhaps even to vaccination in the future. But as long as these host factors remain undefined I think the only thing we can do is – as Dr. Tuyns said – to identify the risk factors, that are those factors which increase the probability that an individual exposed to them will develop a tumour. Our knowledge is still insufficient to point out which of these individuals will develop a tumour and, therefore, this in consequence leads to a preventive strategy. The only preventive strategy which can be adopted is the following: we must decrease the exposure of the total population to these factors because we cannot identify which ones will develop a tumour. You are right in saying that many people who smoke are actually not going to develop a tumour. Life would be much easier for epidemiologists if we were able to say, if you smoke you develop a tumour; but it's not like that.

Kleinsasser: Does somebody else from the panel want to make some additional comments? Then I have to ask the auditory if there are any questions?

Colman (Oxford): I refer especially to the paper of Dr. Schroeder. We had an interest in nasal adenocarcinoma in the Oxford area at one time. I think credit has been given to E. Hadfield (you mentioned her name) who first became aware of this problem and this was taken up later by Macbeth and by Acheson though both of the publications have been by Acheson et al. Although it was realized that all workers in the wood industry were in danger, especially the furniture makers, it's namely the furniture makers that are involved in the polishing process. Possibly the polishing produces a partial burning of the dust but this has been quite uncertain. The instance in the series of adenocarcinoma has been falling dramatically. Not so long ago the adenocarcinoma group constituted 50% of our cases of nasal cancer. But with the improvement of dust extraction the incidence began to fall and I think now it's about only 5–10%. Another attempt was made to improve our identification of these patients or these workers by offering an examination of the nose every 12 months. This has been very unproductive indeed. In the 15 years that this program has been in operation not a single early case has been diagnosed by this method. So it looks as if the diminishing instance is purely resulting from improved dust extraction.

Schroeder: I think it's not so easy to compare the conditions between the two countries (Germany and England). I think there are different working conditions and in our series we did not see only those woodworkers from the furniture industry, but also others, I mentioned coopers, cartwrights, parquet floor layers; these are quite different occupations, and so I think this is a different condition. I'm sorry that I cannot give any data of the incidence because we have not such a small region like High Wycombe – it's a very nice region for observation of such interesting questions. In Germany the whole number of the exposed persons is not quite known, what number of persons are at risk I cannot say. So we can't give the exact data of the incidence rate. The other thing is the prevention or the examination aiming at the detection of early cancer stages. Now we try to find the way in which we can solve this question. We send up some physicians to those workshops, into the industry, to examine those people at their place of work. But till now we did not find any case of cancer; however, the study is still going on.

Jensen: I think I have a few comments to make: First the risk of adenocarcinoma is of course very much increased and very high for wood dust-exposed workers. I was quite interested in your comments that other things may be important like solvents and lacquer. I think these observations are important since the process or the actual carcinogen – if it's not wood dust itself – is really as far as I know not very well described. As you mentioned burning, heat etc. may be important. I have another comment. I was quite surprised that in all of the Federal Republic of Germany over a 12-year period you only had 68 cases recognized as occupationally induced cancer. You must have missed a lot of cases. We had just looked at that in Denmark. It's a country that's about 10 times smaller than the FRG and we have looked very much in detail and so we found many more cases. We had about 40 or 50 cases all together per year of which quite a few are adenocarcinoma cases. And with our recording system we compared that with the cancer registry for adenocarcinomas of the nasal cavities. And even if we have a rather good recording system it's a legal requirement to report cases whenever a position is suspicious that an occupational factor may be involved. Even if that has been a requirement since the mid-1980s it is still so that we could demonstrate that as many cases in addition have had wood dust exposure but had never been reported as an occupational disease for compensation. So I would state that this is true in many countries including the FRG. What you are reporting is really just the top of the iceberg which is what we have seen and I think clinicians should be very much aware of it.

Kleinsasser: I am also a little bit involved in this study as well, but I have to emphasize that not all adenocarcinomas of the nose are wood dust induced. Other ones develop from the mucosal glands and have nothing to do with wood dust.

Schroeder: I did try to get the official data from the insurance institute. It's right what you did say, there might be a lot more cases but only those cases that were diagnosed after 1981 had been recognized legally, so we have missed other cases of wood dust. But I think now this problem is better known and we will have more cases accepted by the insurance institute.

Kleinsasser: Who would like to go on this discussion?

Kraijna (Zagreb): I would like to thank you Mr. Chairman for this excellent conference. I have one simple question: How do you evaluate the inflammation in the ENT organs as a factor promoting carcinogenesis? I know from German statistics for example that you could not find any carcinoma in the mesopharynx after tonsillectomy.

Kleinsasser: We never do evaluate inflammation in carcinogenesis.

de Villiers: I'm not a clinician but as far as the scientific and basic part is concerned I think one has to look at what causes the inflammation and which bacteria or whatever is involved and what the metabolic products of these bacteria are and these could act as carcinogens on certain host-specific cells and then inactivate some factors.

Maran (Edinburgh): Two questions for Dr. de Villier: (1) Does the length of time that the specimen remains in formalin significantly affect the yield of HPV imaging? (2) In situ hybridization: after you insert the probe to the specimen does the number of times you then wash significantly effect the yield of HPV?

de Villiers: To the first question. It depends on the type of fixation whether we can extract because we do all our tests via DNA hybridization and the DNA has to be intact if we extract it from the cells and it is very difficult from formalin-fixed tissues to extract intact DNA. Most of the DNA are degraded and you cannot see the specific sizes of the different bands that we show up by radiolabel probes. It has been proven or shown that for example in oesophageal biopsies which are generally very small, if you use other fixatives than formalin it is easier to obtain the intact DNA. But normally we would like the biopsies for example after being frozen immediately at -17 or $-20\,°C$ and in that way we could do most of the studies on it. With respect to the in situ hybridization which you have mentioned, I have to say that we do not do it in our laboratory because we do not find it is specific enough, so I do not know exactly the procedure, I just know that the whole procedure is very insensitive. There are other procedures where you can show one genome copy or even less than one genome copy per cell in which you cannot do an in situ hybridization. Most of the people involved in the field would tell you that the ideal way of determining the presence of these viruses is by using at least two different techniques: That is combining in situ hybridization with other techniques because you cannot distinguish between some of these virus types. You can say papilloma virus DNA but you cannot say if 1611 or 1618 under some of the conditions that have been used with the in situ hybridization. So you have to determine to use other techniques to specifically determine the type of the virus.

Kleinsasser: I am afraid time is up and so this interesting discussion has to be closed. I should like to thank the panel for their excellent contributions and the audience for their interest and patience.

Subject Index